Massage Works – the Proof

A Compendium of 150 Peer Reviewed Research Studies on the Treatment of 80 Ailments

Volume 1

By Butch Phelps, LMT, AIS & Dr. Harvey Kaltsas, Acupuncture Physician

Copyright 2012 by Butch Phelps, LMT, AIS and Dr. Harvey Kaltsas, AP, Dipl. Ac. (NCCAOM)

Table of Contents

Introduction, 6
Preface, 8
Aggression, 19
Alzheimer's Disease, 19
Ankylosing Spondylitis, 20
Anorexia Nervosa, 20
Anxiety, 21
Atopic Dermatitis, 22
Autism, 22
Blood Pressure, 23
Breast Cancer, 25
Breast Massage, 27
Bulimia, 29
Burn Victims, 30
Cancer, 31
Cardiovascular, 33
Carpal Tunnel Syndrome, 34
Cerebral Palsy, 35
Childhood Anxiety, 36
Childhood Cancer, 36
Chronic Neck Pain, 37
Chronic Shoulder Pain, 38
Depression and Adjustment Disorder, 38

Diabetes, Juvenile, 39
  Employee Anxiety, 40
  Exercise and Massage, 40
  Fibromyalgia, 42
  Gastric Motility in Premature Infants, 44
  Hand Pain, 44
  Headaches, 45
  Herniated Discs, 46
  HIV/AIDS, 47
  Hypertension, 47
  Immune System, 48
  Infants with Colic, 49
  Job Stress, 49
  Labor Pain, 50
  Leukemia, 51
  Lower Back Pain, 51
  Lymph Node Dissection Surgery, 55
  Migraines, 55
  Multiple Sclerosis, 56
  Nausea, 57
  Nervous System, 59
  Neuropathy, 60
  Osgood-Schlatter Disease, 61
  Osteoarthritis, 62
  Oxytocin Levels, 63
  Pain, 64

Parkinson's Disease, 73
Patellafemoral Pain Syndrome –
    PFPS (Runner's Knee), 74
Perineal Massage, 76
Peripheral Neuropathy, 77
Physicians' Perspectives, 78
Physiological Responses to Massage, 78
Plantar Fasciitis, 80
Posttraumatic Stress, 81
Pregnancy, 82
Premature births, 88
Premenstrual Syndrome, 89
Preschool Massage, 90
Preterm Infants, 91
Pulmonary Disease, 101
Renal Disease, 102
Respiratory Infections, 103
Restless Leg Syndrome, 103
Rheumatoid Arthritis, 105
Rotator Cuff Injuries, 106
Sexual Abuse, 107
Sleep, 108
Smoking, 109
Spinal Cord Injuries, 110
Stress, 111
Stroke, 112

Surgery, 113
Tennis Elbow, 114
Thumb and Trigger Finger Pain, 115
TMJ, 116
Torticollis, 116
Transplants, 118
Vagal Activity, 118
Voice Disorders, 119
Whiplash – Mechanical Neck
  Disorders, 120
Afterword, 122
About the Authors, 124

Introduction

From time immemorial, across cultures and continents, massage has been an essential and effective tool used to restore health. Today America faces a crisis in health care costs, yet massage has been largely overlooked and too often is not covered by insurance plans. Regrettably, Medicare does not even include massage therapists as providers. As a result, patients must often turn to more expensive, more invasive, and often less beneficial modes of health care to address their ailments.

Derek Bok, Past President of Harvard University, once said: "If you think education is expensive, try ignorance."

This also applies to the public's lack of awareness as to the benefits of massage therapy, despite the copious amounts of research published in peer-reviewed medical journals as to the efficacy of massage. Sadly, our ignorance is costing us.

This book is a compendium of 150 such peer-reviewed studies on the ability of massage to treat 80 different disorders. We hope therapists will use this research to communicate the benefits of massage to their patients and communities at large. We also hope legislators will read it and pass laws to include massage therapists as providers in federal and state insurance plans, plans which currently only provide for the more expensive types of health care.

In addition, we hope the following preface from Butch Phelps, LMT (Licensed Massage Therapist), AIS (Certified Active Isolated Stretching Therapist) will provide some anecdotal understanding of the benefits of massage from a clinician's perspective.

We are currently working on Volume 2, as more and more research is being completed on the benefits of massage, virtually on a monthly basis.

Dr. Harvey Kaltsas, Acupuncture Physician,
Dipl. Ac. (NCCAOM)

PREFACE

For years the practice of massage therapy in the United States has been looked upon as a luxury. When we think of getting a massage, we typically think of being in a spa and falling asleep while receiving a Swedish massage, which is only one of 224 different types of massage practiced around the world. Swedish, Deep Tissue, and maybe Reflexology are the most popular massage therapies practiced in America. Most people believe that a massage should not be painful. However when there are parts of the body that are stagnant from lack of exercise, over-exercising, and filled with toxins, some massages can be painful because the massage literally moves fluids through the body. Since massage therapy can move fluids within your body, you must fill out an intake form to alert your therapist of any problems you may have, especially if you suffer from blood clots or low blood pressure.

Massage therapy should be looked at as a medical modality, no different than physical therapy or chiropractic. It is the manipulation of the muscles. I prefer to call what I do, "Muscleology." Muscleology is the study of muscles just like Neurology is the study of nerves, cardiology is the study of the heart. There is no college that just studies the muscles of the human body. What is ironic is that 80-90% of our common aches and pains are a result of our muscles tightening or shortening due to activities or lack of activities in our daily lives.

We have tried everything to stop our pains. We have taken pills, undergone injections, and worn braces, pads, lifts, special shoes, or bands. We have even gone as far as surgery trying to correct problems that will come back just simply because we are alive. One just cannot stop the experience of the human condition. Pain is an inevitable byproduct of human activity. It is not optional. But suffering is. Massage offers us a chance to relieve our pains in a healthy, non-toxic manner. It doesn't simply mask the symptoms of pain and provoke long term negative side effects. It can address the underlying root causes of most types of muscle pain.

For years I have been told that plantar fasciitis, the pins and needles sensation you can feel in your heel every morning when getting out of bed, would take from six months to a year to heal, and there is nothing you can about it. Yet by understanding the mechanics of the foot and calf, on a regular basis I have been able to teach people - even by telephone - how to stop their plantar fasciitis within one to two weeks. Western medicine has been trained to go to the point of pain, which would be the heel. Unfortunately, you can numb the pain, but that is not the cause. The cause is in the upper calf just below the knee. Plantar Fasciitis is the result of walking on your toes, running on your toes, playing tennis on your toes, or wearing high heels. Once you understand the cause, fix it, and stop doing the activity that will make it re-occur, you can stop it once and for all. Deep tissue massage and Active Isolated Stretching are the best ways of which I know to stop plantar fasciitis.

As a massage therapist, I combine deep tissue massage and Active isolated Stretching (AIS) to resolve many aches and pains my clients encounter. AIS was founded by Aaron Mattes, who for the last 35 years has written several books about AIS and given seminars all over the world to therapists and physicians. The technique is used by many Olympic athletes.

The way most people stretch is not very effective. Typically, we stretch by holding the stretch for 20-30 seconds, maybe longer. In essence, we are forcing the muscle to elongate. This sets off the stretch reflex, or myotatic reflex, which is in place in all our muscles to prevent us from overstretching our muscles. By stretching the muscles for a prolonged period of time, we initiate the stretch or myotatic reflex, and the muscle contracts to protect us. So we are fighting with our own muscles, and that makes it very difficult for anyone to become more flexible.

Instead, holding a stretch for 2-3 seconds and repeating the stretch 10 times allows the muscle tissue to warm up and expand. This will not set off the stretch reflex, and the muscle becomes more relaxed. By getting the muscles to relax, we can increase the spacing in our joints, allow for better blood flow, and improve nerve conduction. Once the joints have adequate spacing and can move through their full ranges of motion, the joints will lubricate themselves and become healthier. AIS alone could reduce the amount of joint replacements by 30-40%. Obesity is another factor which stresses the joints and necessitates joint replacement, a factor each of us has the ability to get under control to further reduce the need to replace joints.

Pinched nerves, bulging discs, and even herniated discs are caused by unbalanced muscles. Take a look at the spine for example. Between each vertebra is a rubbery disc that acts as a shock absorber. You have a muscle on each side of your spine, the erector spinae that connects at the base of your skull and runs to the top of your pelvis. As the body becomes unbalanced, your spine starts to shift from one side or the other. This will cause an imbalance in the vertebrae and can cause the vertebrae to hit the disc at an angle. Any slight movement in this position could leave you with a bulging disc. Straighten and relax the muscles of the back, and chances are you can relieve the pain.

What we do not know about the muscles of our bodies is killing us, or at the least costing us a fortune. In our research to create this book, we were surprised by the many conditions for which massage therapy is effective. However, there are many ailments for which there is no published research on the efficacy of massage therapy, including several with which I have had personal experience. Among those ailments are breast tenderness, lumps, and even cancer.

I have worked with several women who had complained about breast tenderness and soreness. The women had said their gynecologists told them the soreness was normal. To some degree the doctors were correct; however there are massage options to keep the soreness away. I have seen weekly breast massage reduce the soreness and even take it away. It is amazing how a woman can feel severe pain when first massaging her own breasts, then within minutes feel no pain at all. After doing the weekly massages on themselves, the women reported little to no pain.

Unlike other parts of a woman's body, the breasts have no muscle to push toxins through the fatty tissue of the breast. The movement of the breast as a woman walks will naturally massage her breasts; however, because most women wear bras for a large part of the day, their breasts are stagnant most of the day. Therefore the toxins stay in the fatty tissue, and without weekly self massaging, the breasts can become tender.

Two women came to me with fibrocystic lumps in their breasts that were detected by mammograms and palpated by their physicians. After two months of weekly breast massages, the women went back to their physicians for follow-up mammograms. Neither the mammograms nor the physicians could find the lumps. In fact, one woman said her doctor could not believe the reduction in the density of her breasts. The lumps were gone, and over the last 6-8 months the lumps have not returned. I would love to see some official studies done in this area to see if they get the same results consistently.

I treated one woman who had undergone radiation to kill cancer in her breast. The radiation was successful in killing the cancer, but it had burned her skin. The skin felt like plastic, and her skin, including her breast, had no feeling. The range of motion of her arm was very limited. Over the next 2-3 months I did massage on her chest and breast twice a week. I also did Active Isolated Stretching on her arm and shoulder during the sessions. Over the course of the treatment the feeling returned in her chest and most of her breast, and her arm returned to 90% of her full range of motion. Again, I believe this is an area where massage therapy can become very important for women's health.

The reason for the success in these women's issues is because massage therapy literally moves fluids through the tissue of the human body. As we use our muscles, they consume nutrients in order to hold the contractions. After consuming the nutrients, the muscles leave a waste product called lactic acid. The lactic acid builds up within the muscle tissue and literally blocks some of the blood flow, thereby reducing the body's ability to send the proper amount of oxygen throughout the body. This blockage will cause the muscles to inflame and become tender. Try rubbing the outside of your thighs after a workout or run and chances are they will be tender. The reason for the tenderness is the lactic acid build-up. Understanding massage will allow you to reduce the pain and allow your body to recover faster and remain healthier as you work out.

Your muscles should feel firm, but soft. "Hard Bodies" ®™ is an advertising ploy used to sell a product. "Buns of Steel"®™ is another product that has caused many people to believe their hips should be so hard there is no movement in their hips when they walk. If your hips are that hard, chances are you'll be dealing with low back pain or knee pain.

Too many movies portray bad guys with rock hard bodies and women that never shake or jiggle when they walk. The fact is, your hips and calves should jiggle, not be flabby, when you walk. Most low back pain is a result of rock hard thighs, hips, and even calves. While strength training is a must for a healthy body, stretching and massage are equally as important.

Massage has been practiced as a healing art for thousands of years. Unlike in Asia and Europe, in America massage therapy is not looked upon as a medical treatment. Even the way we train massage therapists is more of a spa training vs. a medical training. Many countries require that massage therapists have a 4 year degree and intern at hospitals working alongside doctors and nurses. Massage therapy can actually help the doctor's treatment work more effectively by opening the blood passages in the muscle tissue which carries the medication throughout your body. When this occurs, patients may need less medication, and their recovery times may be faster.

Massage is not just a luxury. In times of illness it can be a necessity, because it can actually be one of the best ways to help your body heal itself. I have personally seen some amazing results for back pain, headaches, neck and shoulder pain, foot pain, and hand pain. If you get a deep tissue massage at least twice a month, you can eliminate many of your aches and pains. The rejuvenating effects of a proper massage can be the difference between a lifetime of suffering and a lifetime of enjoyment.

Butch Phelps, LMT, AIS

PLEASE NOTE: Some web links cited in this book may have become unavailable since publication, a situation over which we authors unfortunately have no control.

BP
HK

Aggression

1. Web link:
http://www.ncbi.nlm.nih.gov/pubmed/12458696
Journal: *Adolescence. 2002 Fall;37(147):597-607.*
Title: Aggressive adolescents benefit from massage therapy
Authors: Diego MA, Field T, Hernandez-Reif M, Shaw JA, Rothe EM, Castellanos D, Mesner L.
Conclusions: Massage therapy has been shown to reduce aggression. As this study clearly shows by comparison, massage therapy reduces anxiety, hostility, and even other people notice a difference.

Alzheimer's Disease

2. Web link:
http://www.ncbi.nlm.nih.gov/pubmed/10603811
Journal: *J Gerontol Nurs. 1999 Jun;25(6):22-34-*
Title: The effectiveness of slow-stroke massage in diffusing agitated behaviors in individuals with Alzheimer's disease.
Authors: Rowe M, Alfred D.
Conclusions: This study showed that physical agitation was decreased by the slow stroke massage even though verbal agitation did not change.

Ankylosing Spondylitis

3. Web link: http://www.ijtmb.org/index.php/ijtmb/article/view/118
Journal: *International Journal of Therapeutic Massage & Bodywork: Research, Education, & Practice, Vol 4, No 1 (2011)*
Title: The Effects of Massage on Pain, Stiffness, and Fatigue Levels Associated with Ankylosing Spondylitis: A Case Study
Authors: *Rosemary Chunco, LMT, BA, MSc*
Conclusions: This study shows that massage can improve stiffness intensity, duration of stiffness, pain, fatigue and flexion, both lateral and forward. Although there were improvements from the affects of Ankylosing Spondylitis, further studies need to be performed to validate these findings.

Anorexia Nervosa

4. Web link: http://www6.miami.edu/touch-research/AdultMassage.html
Journal: Touch Research Institute
Title: Anorexia
Authors: Hart, S., Field, T., Hernandez-Reif, M., Nearing, G., Shaw, S., Schanberg, S. & Kuhn, C. (2001).
Conclusions: Massage therapy reduced the anxiety levels immediately. Over the time of the study massage therapy reduced cortisol levels and increased dopamine and norepinephrine levels.

Anxiety

5. Web link:
http://www.ncbi.nlm.nih.gov/pubmed/20347840
Journal: *Complement Ther Clin Pract. 2010 May;16(2):92-5. Epub 2009 Nov 14.*
Title: Effect of massage therapy on pain, anxiety, and tension in cardiac surgical patients: a pilot study
Authors: Cutshall SM, Wentworth LJ, Engen D, Sundt TM, Kelly RF, Bauer BA.
Conclusions: In this study two groups of patients undergoing cardiac surgery were used. The massaged group showed significant reduction in pain, anxiety, and tension when compared to the group that did not receive massage.

6. Web link:
http://www.ncbi.nlm.nih.gov/pubmed/20347836
Journal: *Complement Ther Clin Pract. 2010 May;16(2):70-5. Epub 2009 Jul 14.*
Title: Effect of massage therapy on pain, anxiety, and tension after cardiac surgery: a randomized study.
Authors: Bauer BA, Cutshall SM, Wentworth LJ, Engen D, Messner PK, Wood CM, Brekke KM, Kelly RF, Sundt TM 3rd.
Conclusions: In this study patients were divided into 2 groups, either massage or relaxation. The massage group showed significant reductions in pain, anxiety, and tension compared to the relaxation group.

Atopic Dermatitis

7. Web link:
http://www.ncbi.nlm.nih.gov/pubmed/9796594
Journal: *Pediatric Dermatology, 15*, 390-395.
Title: Atopic dermatitis symptoms decreased in children following massage therapy
Authors: Schachner, L., Field, T., Hernandez-Reif, M., Duarte, A. & Krasnegor, J. (1998)
Conclusions: In this study, after 1 month of massage therapy, the massaged group of children had significant reductions in anxiety, redness, scaling, lichenification, excoriation, and pruritus. The non-massaged group only had reduction in scaling. This study shows that massage therapy may be a cost effective treatment for Atopic Dermatitis.

Autism

8. Web link: http://www6.miami.edu/touch-research/Massage.html
Journal: *Journal of Autism and Developmental Disorders, 27*, 329-334.
Title: Autistic children's attentiveness and responsivity improved after touch therapy
Authors: Field, T., Lasko, D., Mundy, P., Henteleff, T., Talpins, S., & Dowling, M. (1986).
Conclusions: In this study, the massage therapy group showed a reduction in touch aversion, off task behavior, irrelevant sounds, and stereotypic behaviors.

9. Web link: http://www6.miami.edu/touch-research/ChildMassage.html
Journal: *Journal of Autism and Developmental Disorders, 31,* 513-516.
Title: Improvements in the behavior of children with autism
Authors: Escalona, A., Field, T., Singer-Strunk, R., Cullen, C., & Hartshorn, K. (2001).
Conclusions: This study lasted for 1 month and it divided children into a reading group and a massage group. The massage group had reductions in stereotypic behaviors, off task behaviors, and better social skills during play.

Blood Pressure

10. Web link:
http://www.ncbi.nlm.nih.gov/pubmed/16494570
Journal: *Journal of Alternative and Complementary Medicine.* 2006 Jan-Feb;12(1):65-70.
Title: Changes in blood pressure after various forms of therapeutic massage: a preliminary study.
Authors: Cambron JA, Dexheimer J, Coe P.
Conclusions: 150 adults with a blood pressure under 150/95 were given randomly Swedish massage, trigger point massage, and sports massage. Their blood pressure was tested before and after the massage. The participants were grouped based on age, height, and type of massage. Overall the systolic blood pressure

decreased slightly and the diastolic blood pressure increased slightly on average. Swedish massage had the greatest impact as it reduced the systolic and diastolic blood pressure. The Trigger point increased the systolic blood pressure. If both Trigger point and sports massage were used during a session, then the diastolic pressure increased as well. The deeper the massage the higher the increase of blood pressure.

11. Web link:
http://www.ncbi.nlm.nih.gov/pubmed/17654092
Journal: *International Journal Neuroscience. 2007 Sep;117(9):1281-7.*
Title: Effects of aromatherapy massage on blood pressure and lipid profile in Korean climacteric women.
Authors: Hur MH, Oh H, Lee MS, Kim C, Choi AN, Shin GR.
Conclusions: 58 menopausal women were divided into two groups: 30 women were in the aromatherapy massage group and 28 women were in the control group. The massage group received a 30 minute massage once a week for 2- 8 week periods as well self abdominal massage at home. The massage used lavender, rose geranium, rose, and jasmine. Both groups were tested before and after the study. There were significant improvements on systolic and diastolic blood pressures in both groups.

12. Web link: http://www6.miami.edu/touch-research/AdultMassage.html
Journal: *Journal of Bodywork and Movement Therapies,*

4, 31-38.
Title: High blood pressure and associated symptoms were reduced by massage therapy
Authors: Hernandez-Reif, M., Field, T., Krasnegor, J. & Theakston, H.(2000)
Conclusions: High blood pressure is associated with elevated anxiety, stress and stress hormones, hostility, depression and catecholamines. Massage therapy and progressive muscle relaxation were evaluated as treatments for reducing blood pressure and these associated symptoms. Diagnosed Hypertensive adults received ten 30 minute massage sessions over five weeks or they were given progressive muscle relaxation instructions. Sitting diastolic blood pressure decreased after the first and last massage therapy sessions and reclining diastolic blood pressure decreased from the first to the last day of the study. Although both groups reported less anxiety, only the massage therapy group reported less depression and hostility and showed decreased cortisol. This study shows that massage therapy has a definite affect on several of the causes of hypertension.

Breast Cancer

13. Web link:
http://www.ncbi.nlm.nih.gov/pubmed/19388859
Journal: *J Altern Complement Med. 2009 Apr;15(4):373-80.*
Title: Effects of therapeutic massage on the quality of life among patients with breast cancer during treatment

Authors: Sturgeon M, Wetta-Hall R, Hart T, Good M, Dakhil S.
Conclusions: In this study each patient was given a 30 minute breast massage each week for 3 weeks. After 3 weeks results showed reduction in pain, nausea, sleep quality, and quality of life symptoms, although the reduction was not significant.

14. Web link:
http://www.sciencedirect.com/science/article/pii/S156607020900085X
Journal: *Autonomic Neuroscience Volume 150, Issues 1-2, 5 October 2009, Pages 111-115*
Title: The effect of massage on immune function and stress in women with breast cancer — A randomized controlled trial
Authors: A. Billhult, C. Lindholm, Ronny Gunnarsson, and E. Stener-Victorin,
Conclusions: This study showed that 1 full-body light pressure effleurage massage can reduce the deterioration of peripheral blood natural killer cell activity, reduce heart rate, and reduce systolic blood pressure for the short term. It had no effect on cortisol levels or diastolic blood pressure. However the long term effects need to be further investigated.

15. Web link:
http://www.ncbi.nlm.nih.gov/pubmed/15809216
Journal: *Int J Neurosci. 2005 Apr;115(4):495-510.*
Title: Natural killer cells and lymphocytes increase in women with breast cancer following massage therapy

Authors: Hernandez-Reif M, Field T, Ironson G, Beutler J, Vera Y, Hurley J, Fletcher MA, Schanberg S, Kuhn C, Fraser M.
Conclusions: In this study, women were divided into 2 groups:
   1. massage therapy (or progressive muscle relaxation) for 30-minute sessions 3 times per week for 5 weeks or
   2. standard treatment.
The massaged group reported less anger, depression, and more energy. The massage therapy group showed increases in Dopamine levels, Natural killer cells, and lymphocytes from first to last day of the study.

16. Web link:
http://www.ncbi.nlm.nih.gov/pubmed/10660924
Journal: *Oncol Nurs Forum. 2000 Jan-Feb;27(1):67-72.*
Title: The effects of foot reflexology on anxiety and pain in patients with breast and lung cancer
Authors: Stephenson NL, Weinrich SP, Tavakoli AS.
Conclusions: Patients suffering from breast cancer and lung cancer were given reflexology (foot massages) for just 30 minutes. Each of the patients reported a decrease in anxiety, and the breast cancer patients showed decrease in pain according to one of three pain measures.

Breast Massage

17. Web link:
http://www.ncbi.nlm.nih.gov/pubmed/15097435

Journal: *Journal of Pediatric Gastroenterology and Nutrition. 2004 May;38(5):484-7.*
Title: Composition of milk obtained from unmassaged versus massaged breasts of lactating mothers.
Authors: Foda, M.I., Kawashima, T., Nakamura, S., Kobayashi, M., & Oku, T. (2004)
Conclusions: Using two sets of milk samples at two different periods, Oketani breast massage caused a significant increase in the lipids, especially in the second sample. Total solids increased from the first day to 11 months postpartum. Finally breast massage may improve the growth and the development of infants.

18. Web link:
http://banglajol.info/index.php/JBCPS/article/download/4293/3535
Journal: *Journal of Bangladesh College of Physical Surgery 2009; 27: 155-159)*
Title: Oketani Lactation Management: A New Method to Augment Breast Milk
Authors: N KABIR, S TASNIM
Conclusions: Using the Oketani breast massage improves the venous blood flow of the breast tissue, removes the adhesions of breast tissue to the pectoralis major muscle (Chest muscle), frees the milk ducts, and improves the softness and health of the nipple. Oketani breast massage helps to prevent inverted nipples and nipple soreness, while improving milk production.

19. Web link:
http://www.ncbi.nlm.nih.gov/pubmed/21964220

Journal: *Journal of Korean Academic Nursing. 2011 Aug;41(4):451-9. doi: 10.4040/jkan.2011.41.4.451.*
Title: Effects of Breast Massage on Breast Pain, Breast-milk Sodium, and Newborn Suckling in Early Postpartum Mothers
Authors: Ahn S, Kim J, Cho J.
Conclusions: 60 postpartum mothers that were having trouble breast feeding participated in this study. The massage group received two 30 minute breast massages within a 10 day period and the control group received routine care. After the first massage, the mothers reported a reduction in breast pain, increase in the babies suckling, and a reduction in breast milk sodium. Breast massage can relieve painful breasts, lower the sodium in breast milk and improve suckling from the babies. Regular breast massage is very beneficial for maintaining healthier breasts.

Bulimia

20. Web link: http://www6.miami.edu/touch-research/ChildMassage.html
Journal: *Adolescence, 33,* 555-563
Title: Bulimic adolescents benefit from massage therapy
Authors: Field, T., Schanberg, S., Kuhn, C., Fierro, K., Henteleff, T., Mueller, C., Yando, R., & Burman, I. (1998)
Conclusions: In this study the patients receiving massage therapy showed lower anxiety levels, depression levels, cortisol levels, and higher dopamine levels.

Burn Victims

21. Web link:
http://www.ncbi.nlm.nih.gov/pubmed/20453734
Journal: *Journal of Burn Care Residency. 2010 May-Jun;31(3):429-32.*
Title: Itching, pain, and anxiety levels are reduced with massage therapy in burned adolescents
Authors: Parlak Gürol A, Polat S, Akçay MN
Conclusions: During the study, the patients receiving massage therapy experienced reduced pain, itching, and anxiety. In most cultures massage therapy is used to reduce a wide range of burn symptoms.

22. Web link:
http://www.ncbi.nlm.nih.gov/pubmed/10850898
Journal: *J Burn Care Rehabil. 2000 May-Jun;21(3):189-93.*
Title: Postburn itching, pain, and psychological symptoms are reduced with massage therapy
Authors: Field T, Peck M, Scd, Hernandez-Reif M, Krugman S, Burman I, Ozment-Schenck
Conclusions: After 5 weeks of massage therapy to moderate size scar tissue, the patients reported a reduction of pain, itching, and anxiety. Their moods improved immediately.

Cancer

23. Web link:
http://www.ncbi.nlm.nih.gov/pubmed/10660924
Journal: *Oncol Nurs Forum. 2000 Jan-Feb;27(1):67-72.*
Title: The effects of foot reflexology on anxiety and pain in patients with breast and lung cancer
Authors: Stephenson NL, Weinrich SP, Tavakoli AS.
Conclusions: Patients suffering from breast cancer and lung cancer were given reflexology(foot massages) for just 30 minutes. Each of the patients reported a decrease in anxiety, and the breast cancer patients showed a reduction in one of the three pain measures.

24. Web link:
http://www.ncbi.nlm.nih.gov/pubmed/10851775
Journal: *Cancer Nurs. 2000 Jun;23(3):237-43.*
Title: Foot massage. A nursing intervention to modify the distressing symptoms of pain and nausea in patients hospitalized with cancer.
Authors: Grealish L, Lomasney A, Whiteman B
Conclusions: Cancer patients were given a 10 minute foot massage (5 minutes per foot). The foot massage had a significant effect on the perceptions of pain, nausea, and relaxation when measured on a visual analog scale.

25. Web link:
http://web.me.com/touchmaster/nurture/Clinical_Trials.html

Journal: *Hospice Journal, 15*, 31-53
Title: Effects of massage on pain intensity, analgesics and quality of life in patients with cancer pain: A pilot study of a randomized clinical trial conducted within hospice care delivery.
Authors: Wilkie, D.J.; Kampbell, J.; Cutshall, S.; Halabisky, H.; Harmon, H.; Johnson, L.P.; Weinacht, L.; & Rake-Marona, M. (2000).
Conclusions: When compared to a group without massage, the pain intensity decreased by 42% vs. 25% without massage. Pulse rate and respiratory rate were significantly reduced as well.

26. Web link:
http://www.ncbi.nlm.nih.gov/pubmed/12237988
Journal: *Journal of Nurse Scholarships. 2002;34(3):257-62*
Title: Outcomes of therapeutic massage for hospitalized cancer patients
Authors: Smith MC, Kemp J, Hemphill L, Vojir CP
Conclusions: Massage therapy reduced the levels of pain, sleep quality, symptom distress and anxiety. Massage therapy has the potential to be a valuable tool for nurses working with cancer patients.

27. Web link:
http://ict.sagepub.com/content/2/4/332.abstract
Journal: *Integrative Cancer Therapies*
Title: Therapeutic Massage and Healing Touch Improve Symptoms in Cancer
Authors: Janice Post-White, RN, PhD,FAAN, Mary

Ellen Kinney, RN, BA, CHTP, Kay Savik, MS, Joanna Berntsen Gau, RN, MS, Carol Wilcox, RN, MS, Irving Lerner, MD

Conclusions: Massage therapy reduces pain, mood disturbances, and fatigue in patients receiving cancer chemotherapy. Less anti-inflammatory drug was needed during the chemotherapy.

28. Web link:
http://nccam.nih.gov/research/results/spotlight/110608.htm
Journal: *Annals of Internal Medicine.* 2008;149(6):369–379.
Title: Massage therapy versus simple touch to improve pain and mood in patients with advanced cancer: a randomized trial
Authors: Kutner J, Smith M, Corbin S, et al.
Conclusion: 380 patients with advanced cancer and suffering from moderate to severe pain were used in this study. 90% were in hospice care. Each patient was given six 30 minute massages or simple touch sessions daily for 2 weeks. The conclusion of the study showed that massage gave immediate relief initially. Over the period of the study both massage and simple touch reduced pain and anxiety. The study also suggested that simple touch from family may be helpful to the comfort of the patient.

Cardiovascular

29. Web link:
http://www.ncbi.nlm.nih.gov/pubmed/20002340

Journal: *Prog Cardiovasc Nurs. 2009 Dec;24(4):155-61.*
Title: Massage therapy reduces tension, anxiety, and pain in patients awaiting invasive cardiovascular procedures.
Authors: Wentworth LJ, Briese LJ, Timimi FK, Sanvick CL, Bartel DC, Cutshall SM, Tilbury RT, Lennon R, Bauer BA
Conclusion: Patients undergoing cardiovascular procedures reported an increase in satisfaction when they were given a 20 minute massage prior to the procedure vs. patients that did not receive a massage. The massaged patients reported an improvement in anxiety, tension, and pain.

Carpal Tunnel Syndrome

30. Web link:
http://www.massagetherapyfoundation.org/pdf/Massage%20and%20carpal%20tunnel%20syndrome.pdf
Journal: *Journal of Bodywork and Movement Therapies*, 8, 9-14.
Title: Carpal tunnel syndrome symptoms are lessened following massage therapy.
Authors: Field, T., Diego, Miguel, Cullen, Christy, Hartshorn, Kristin, Gruskin, Alan, Hernandez-Reif, Maria, Sunshine, William.
Conclusions: The massage therapy group, when compared to a group without massage, showed greater improvement in grip strength, pain, anxiety, and depression. The massage group had improvements on

the nerve conduction.

31. Web link:
http://www.sciencedirect.com/science/article/pii/S1360859203000640
Journal: *Journal of Bodywork and Movement Therapies*
Title: Carpal tunnel syndrome symptoms are lessened following massage therapy.
Authors: Tiffany Field, Miguel Diego, Christy Cullen, Kristin Hartshorn, Alan Gruskin, Maria Hernandez-Reif and William Sunshine
Conclusions: The massage therapy participants showed improved grip strength and peak latency, while having lower levels of perceived pain, anxiety, and depression. The study shows that daily massage therapy can reduce the symptoms of carpal tunnel syndrome.

Cerebral Palsy

32. Web link:
http://www.kidsmassage.com.au/Cerebral_Palsy_Symptoms_in_Children_Decreased_Following_Massage_Therapy.pdf
Journal: *Early Child Development and Care, 175, 445-456.*
Title: Cerebral palsy symptoms in children decreased following massage therapy.
Authors: Hernandez-Reif, M., Field, T., Largie, S., Diego, M., Manigat, N., Seoanes, M., & Bornstein, J. (2005).

Conclusions: Children suffering from cerebral palsy were massaged twice a week for 30 minutes. The children had reduced spasticity, rigid muscle tone, improved fine and gross motor skills. The massaged children showed more positive facial expressions and less limb activity during face to face play.

Childhood Anxiety

33. Web link: http://www6.miami.edu/touch-research/ChildMassage.html
Journal: *Journal of the American Academy of Child and Adolescent Psychiatry, 31,* 125-131.
Title: Massage reduces anxiety in child and adolescent psychiatric patients.
Authors: Field, T., Morrow, C., Valdeon, C., Larson, S., Kuhn, C., & Schanberg, S., (1992).
Conclusions: Massage therapy lowered their depression, anxiety levels, urinary cortisol, and norepinephrine, while increasing their nighttime sleep. Parents reported a reduction in anxiety levels.

Childhood Cancer

34. Web link:
http://integrativetherapies.columbia.edu/research/mass.html
Journal: *International Journal of Therapeutic Massage & Bodywork.* 2009; (2)2:7-14.
Title: Children with Cancer and Blood Diseases Experience Positive Physical and Psychological Effects

from Massage Therapy
Authors: Haun JN, Graham-Pol J, Shortley B.
Conclusions: 30 children from age 6 months to 17 years were divided into 3 groups. One group received in hospital massage daily, the second group received outpatient massage weekly, and the third group did not get any massages. The massage groups showed significant progress in physical improvements on muscle soreness discomfort, respiratory rate and overall progress. Massage therapy can reduce psychological and physical distress in cancer patients.

Chronic Neck Pain

35. Web link:
http://nccam.nih.gov/research/results/spotlight/051809.htm
Journal: *Clinical Journal of Pain.* 2009;25(3):233–238
Title: Randomized trial of therapeutic massage for chronic neck pain.
Authors: Sherman KJ, Cherkin DC, Hawkes RJ, et al
Conclusions: 64 people suffering with neck pain for at least 12 weeks were chosen randomly to be either in a massage group or a self care book group. The patients were assessed at 4, 10, and 26 weeks. After 4 weeks the massage group had significant increases in range of motion and reduction in pain. At 10 weeks the massage group, compared to the self care book group, had improvements in movements and symptoms. At 26 weeks, the massage group, compared to the self care book group, reported better movement, but about the same on symptoms. At the end of the 26 weeks the self

care book group had increased their medications by 14% whereas the massage group stayed the same. The most improvement came at the 4 week interval for the massage group.

Chronic Shoulder Pain

36. Web link:
http://www.ncbi.nlm.nih.gov/pubmed/19329049
Journal:
J Bodyw Mov Ther. 2009 Apr;13(2):128-35. Epub 2008 Jun 24.
Title: Application of Fascial Manipulation technique in chronic shoulder pain--anatomical basis and clinical implications.
Authors: Day JA, Stecco C, Stecco A.
Conclusions: The use of Fascial Manipulation on 28 patients with chronic posterior brachial pain reduced the pain. Fascial manipulations on the shoulder can be very effective in reducing the pain in chronic shoulder dysfunctions.

Depression and Adjustment Disorder

37. Web link: http://www6.miami.edu/touch-research/ChildMassage.html
Journal: *Journal of the American Academy of Child & Adolescent Psychiatry, 31*, 125-131.
Title: Massage reduces depression and anxiety in child and adolescent psychiatric patients

Authors: Field, T., Morrow, C., Valdeon, C., Larson, S., Kuhn, C., & Schanberg, S.(1992)
Conclusions: 52 Children were divided into 2 groups. One group was given daily massages and the other group watched relaxing videos. The massaged group showed less depression, anxiety, and slept better. The massaged children had lowered saliva cortisol levels, urinary cortisol and norepinephrine levels. The children that watched videos were virtually unchanged.

Diabetes, Juvenile

38. Web link: http://www6.miami.edu/touch-research/ChildMassage.html
Journal: *Diabetes Spectrum ,10*, 237-239.
Title: Massage therapy lowers blood glucose levels in children with diabetes
Authors: Field, T., Hernandez-Reif, M., Larissa A., Shaw, K., Schanberg, S., & Kuhn, C. (1997)
Conclusions: 20 diabetic children were place into 2 groups. One group received daily massages for 30 days, while the second group was given relaxation therapy. The massaged group showed a reduction in parent anxiety and depressed moods. The children showed a reduction in anxiety, fidgetiness and depression. Over the 30 days the blood glucose levels, with proper use of insulin and diet, decreased from 159 to within normal range.

Employee Anxiety

39. Web link:
http://jab.sagepub.com/content/32/2/160.short
Journal: *The Journal of Applied Behavioral Sciences*
Title: The Effectiveness of Massage Therapy Intervention on Reducing Anxiety in the Workplace
Authors: Shulman, K.R. & Jones, G.E. (1996).
Conclusions: 18 employees were divided into 2 groups. One group received chair massage and the other group received Break Therapy. Stress levels were measured, using the State Trait Anxiety Inventory, before and after test as well as a delayed test later. The anxiety levels in the massaged employees were significantly reduced.

Exercise and Massage

40. Web link:
http://bjsm.bmj.com/content/38/2/173.abstract
Journal: *British Journal of Sports Medicine*
Title: Effects of leg massage on recovery from high intensity cycling exercise
Journal: *British Journal of Sports Medicine*
Authors: Robertson, A., Watt, J.M. & Galloway, S.D. (2004)
Conclusions: 9 men were divided into 2 groups, one received leg massages and the other group rested laying down. Each man performed six 30 second high intensity exercises with a 30 second active recovery period

between each exercise. Heart rate, peak power, and mean power were identical. However in the massaged group the fatigued levels were significantly lower.

41. Web link:
http://www.ncbi.nlm.nih.gov/pubmed/12547748
Journal: *Br J Sports Med. 2003 Feb;37(1):72-5*
Title: The Effects of Massage on Delayed Onset Muscle Soreness.
Authors: Hilbert, J.E., Sforzo, G.A. & Swensen, T. (2003)
Conclusions: 18 people were divided into 2 groups, massaged and control groups. Each participant created delayed onset muscle soreness by doing 6 sets of 8 maximal eccentric contractions of the right hamstring followed 2 hours later with a massage for the massaged group. At 2, 6, 24, and 48 hours after the exercises, peak torque, mood range, range of motion, intensity, and degree of soreness were assessed. The degree of soreness in the massaged group was significantly lowered when compared to the non-massaged group.

42. Web link:
http://www.ncbi.nlm.nih.gov/pubmed/18385196
Journal: *British Journal Sports Med. 2008 Oct;42(10):834-8. Epub 2008 Apr 2*
Title: Effects of Petrissage Massage on Fatigue and Exercise Performance Following Intensive Cycle Pedaling.
Authors: Ogai R, Yamane M, Matsumoto T, Kosaka M
Conclusions: 11 young women were divided into 2

groups, a massaged group and a non-massaged group. The women were asked to engage in exercise sessions on the cycle ergometer. The loads were based on the women's weight so the loads would be equal. Lactate levels, muscle stiffness, and fatigue were taken during their 35 minute rest. There were 2 tests with no less than 1 week apart. During the first test there were no significant changes between the groups. During the second test there was significant improvement in muscle stiffness and lower limb fatigue for the massaged group vs. non-massaged group.

Fibromyalgia

43. Web link:
http://www.ncbi.nlm.nih.gov/pubmed/17041326
Journal: *Journal of Clinical Rheumatol. 2002 Apr;8(2):72-6.*
Title: Fibromyalgia pain and substance P decrease and sleep improves after massage therapy.
Authors: Field T, Diego M, Cullen C, Hernandez-Reif M, Sunshine W, Douglas S.
Conclusions: 24 people suffering from fibromyalgia were assigned to either a massage group or a relaxation therapy group. The massaged group got a 30 minute massage twice a week for 5 weeks. During the study both groups showed a decrease in anxiety and depression. However the massaged group had an increase in sleep hours, P levels reduced, and their doctors reported lower disease, pain levels, and less

tender points.

44. Web link:
http://www.ncbi.nlm.nih.gov/pubmed/21234327
Journal: *Evidence Based Complement Alternative Medicine. 2011;2011:561753. Epub 2010 Dec 28.*
Title: Benefits of massage-myofascial release therapy on pain, anxiety, quality of sleep, depression, and quality of life in patients with fibromyalgia.
Authors: Castro-Sánchez AM, Matarán-Peñarrocha GA, Granero-Molina J, Aguilera-Manrique G, Quesada-Rubio JM, Moreno-Lorenzo C.
Conclusions: The purpose of the present study was to determine whether massage-myofascial release therapy can improve pain, anxiety, quality of sleep, depression, and quality of life in patients with fibromyalgia. Seventy-four fibromyalgia patients were randomly assigned to massage-myofascial release therapy or a control group. The study was for 20 weeks. Pain, anxiety, quality of sleep, depression, and quality of life were determined at the beginning of the study, after the last treatment session, and at 1 month and 6 months. For the first month, anxiety levels, quality of sleep, pain, and quality of life were improved in the massage group over the control group. However, at 6 months after the study, there were only significant differences in the quality of sleep index. Myofascial release techniques improved pain and quality of life in patients with fibromyalgia.

Gastric Motility in Premature Infants

45. Web link: http://www.jpeds.com/article/S0022-3476%2805%2900186-1/abstract
Journal: *The Journal of Pediatrics Volume 147, Issue 1, Pages 50-55, July 2005*
Title: Vagal Activity, Gastric Motility, and Weight Gain in Massaged Preterm Neonates
Authors: Diego MA, Field T, Hernandez-Reif M. (2005)
Conclusions: Premature infants were divided into 3 groups, moderate massage, light massage, and no massage. Of the 3 groups only the moderate massage group showed significant increases in weight gain, vagal tone, and gastric motility. Gastric motility and vagal tone were significantly related to weight gain.

Hand Pain

46. Web link:
http://www.ncbi.nlm.nih.gov/pubmed/21982138
Journal: *Complementary Therapy Clinic Practice. 2011 Nov;17(4):226-9. Epub 2011 Mar 15.*
Title: Hand pain is reduced by massage therapy.
Authors: Field T, Diego M, Delgado J, Garcia D, Funk CG.
Conclusions: 46 people were randomly assigned to a massage group and standard treatment group. The massage received a treatment once a week from a therapist and taught to do self massage daily. The massage group had lower pain ratings and better grip

strength than the control group. The massage group also had lower depression and anxiety levels as well.

Headaches

47. Web link:
http://www.ncbi.nlm.nih.gov/pubmed/12356617
Journal: *American Journal of Public Health. 2002 Oct;92(10):1657-61. Volume 147, Issue 1 , Pages 50-55, July 2005*
Title: Massage therapy and frequency of chronic tension headaches
Authors: Quinn C, Chandler C, Moraska A.
Conclusions: 4 people suffering from chronic tension headaches received massage treatment for 4 weeks. Headache frequency, duration, and intensity were measured comparing to the baseline measurement. After the massage treatment the number of headaches and duration were greatly reduced.

48. Weblink:
http://www.sciencedaily.com/releases/2010/07/100708081233.htm
Journal: *ScienceDaily (July 11, 2010)*
Title: Simple Massage Relieves Chronic Tension Headache
Author: Cristina Toro Velasco
Conclusions: Psychological and physiological state of patients with tension headache improves within 24 hours after receiving a 30-minute massage. By massaging

cervical trigger points, the patients' autonomic nervous system improved and the patients showed improved psychological stress with less stress and anxiety. The relief was still evident 24 hours later.

49. Web link:
http://www.ncbi.nlm.nih.gov/pmc/articles/PMC2565109/
Journal: *Journal of Manual Manipulative Therapy. 2008; 16(2): 106–112*
Title: Changes in Clinical Parameters in Patients with Tension-type Headache Following Massage Therapy
Authors: Albert Moraska, PhD and Clint Chandler, BS, LMT
Conclusions: 16 participants were placed in 4 three week phases. The 1st phase was the baseline phase, then 2 massage phases, and a follow up phase. Each participant kept a headache diary daily to record incidence, intensity, and duration. During the massage phases each patient received two 45 minute massages weekly. Reduction in incidence, intensity, and duration occurred in every phase including the follow up.

Herniated Discs

50. Web link:
http://www.ncbi.nlm.nih.gov/pubmed/11272089
Journal: *Prof Inferm. 2000 Apr-Jun;53(2):80-7.*
Title: The effectiveness of foot reflexotherapy on chronic pain associated with a herniated disk
Authors: Degan M, Fabris F, Vanin F, Bevilacqua M, Genova V, Mazzucco M, Negrisolo A

Conclusions: 40 people suffering from lumbar-sacral disc hernia received 3 reflexology treatments for a week. At the end of the study 62.5 % of the people reported a reduction in pain.

HIV/AIDS

51. Web link:
http://www.ncbi.nlm.nih.gov/pubmed/8707483
Journal: *International Journal of Neuroscience. 1996 Feb;84(1-4):205-17*
Title- Massage therapy is associated with enhancement of the immune system's cytotoxic capacity
Authors: Ironson G, Field T, Scafidi F, Hashimoto M, Kumar M, Kumar A, Price A, Goncalves A, Burman I, Tetenman C, Patarca R, Fletcher MA
Conclusions: 29 men received daily massages for one month. Eleven of the men got massages for one month, then a month with no massages; these were the control group. During the month of massage the men had significant increases in Natural Killer Cell number and there were no changes in the HIV disease progression markers. There were decreases in anxiety and increases in relaxation. There appears to be an increase in cytotoxic capacity associated with massage.

Hypertension

52. Web link:
http://brn.sagepub.com/content/7/2/98.abstract

Journal- *Biological Research for Nursing*
Title - The Effect of Therapeutic Back Massage in Hypertensive Persons: A Preliminary Study
Author: Christine M. Olney
Conclusions: Hypertension patients were given a 10 minute back massage 3 times per week for 10 weeks. Both the Systolic and Diastolic blood pressure decreased.

Immune System

53. Web link:
http://nccam.nih.gov/research/results/spotlight/090110.htm
Journal: *The Journal of Alternative and Complementary Medicine.* 2010;16(10):1–10.
Title: Study Examines the Effects of Swedish Massage Therapy on Hormones, Immune Function
Author: Rapaport MH, Schettler P, Bresee C.
Conclusion: 53 adults randomly received a 45 minute Swedish massage or 45 minutes of light touch. Blood samples were taken before and after the sessions. The result was the Swedish massage group had a decrease in the hormone arginine - vasopressin, which regulates blood pressure and water retention, after just one session. The stress cortisol and the lymphocytes were virtually unchanged in both groups. Conclusively it is shown that just one session of Swedish massage can have a significant effect on the biological systems of our bodies.

Infants with Colic

54. Web link:
http://www.ncbi.nlm.nih.gov/pubmed/10835097
Journal: *Pediatrics. 2000 Jun;105(6):E84.*
Title: Infant massage compared with crib vibrator in the treatment of colicky infants.
Authors: Huhtala V, Lehtonen L, Heinonen R, Korvenranta H.
Conclusions: Infants less then 7 weeks old and suffering from colic were placed randomly into 2 groups. One group received massage 3 times a day and the other group receive crib vibration 3 times a day for 4 weeks. Over the 4 weeks the total amount of crying and colicky crying decreased significantly for both groups. Infant massage is comparable to the use of crib vibration in reducing colicky crying in infants.

Job Stress

55. Web link: http://www.stress.org.uk/Research-Results.aspx
Journal: *International Journal of Neuroscience, 86, 197-205.*
Title: Massage therapy reduces anxiety and enhances EEG pattern of alertness and math computations
Authors: Field, T., Ironson, G., Scafidi, F., Nawrocki, T., Goncalves, A., Burman, I., Pickens, J., Fox, N., Schanberg, S., & Kuhn, C. (1996)
Conclusions: 50 people were divided into 2 groups.

Those in first group were given chair massage and those in the second group were asked to relax in a massage chair for 15 minutes 2 times per week for 5 weeks. Before and after each session the participants were ask to perform some math computations, POMS depression, State Anxiety Scales, and provide a saliva sample for cortisol. The study showed that the massage group had more alertness, increased speed and better accuracy on math computations. At the end of the 5 week period the anxiety levels and the job stress score was lower only for the massage group. Both groups reported lower depression.

Labor Pain

56. Web link:
http://www.ncbi.nlm.nih.gov/pubmed/9443139
Journal: *Journal of Psychosomatic Obstetrics and Gynecology. 1997 Dec;18(4):286-91*
Title: Labor pain is reduced by massage therapy.
Authors: Field T, Hernandez-Reif M, Taylor S, Quintino O, Burman I.
Conclusions: Twenty-eight women were randomly placed either
 a) in a group to receive massage in addition to coaching in breathing from their partners during labor or
 b) in a group to receive coaching in breathing alone (a technique learned during prenatal classes).
The massaged mothers reported a decrease in depressed mood, anxiety and pain, and showed less

agitated activity and anxiety. In addition, the massaged mothers had significantly shorter labors, a shorter hospital stay, and less postpartum depression.

Leukemia

57. Web link: http://www6.miami.edu/touch-research/ChildMassage.html
Journal: *Journal of Bodywork and Movement Therapies, 5,* 271-274.
Title: Leukemia immune changes following massage therapy.
Authors: Field, T., Cullen, C., Diego, M., Hernandez-Reif, M., Sprinz, P., Beebe, K., Kissel, B., & Bango-Sanchez, V. (2001)
Conclusions: Twenty children with leukemia were provided with daily massage therapy by their parents and were compared to a standard treatment control group. Following a month of massage therapy, depressed mood decreased in the children's parents, and the children's white blood cell and neutrophil counts decreased.

Lower Back Pain

58. Web link: http://www.jpsmjournal.com/article/S0885-3924(98)00129-8/abstract
Journal: *Journal of Pain and Symptom Management*
Title: Massage Therapy for Low Back Pain
Authors: Edzard Ernst, MD, PhD, FRCP

Conclusions: 4 clinical trails were used and massage therapy was used as a monotherapy. One trial suggested massage was better than no treatment. Two trials suggested massage was no better than Spinal manipulation or Transcutaneous Electrical Stimulation. Finally one trial suggested it was not more effective than spinal manipulation. There are too few trials for massage therapy as a resolution to low back pain. Massage could be a good treatment for low back pain.

59. Web link: http://www6.miami.edu/touch-research/Massage.html
Journal: *CMAJ, 162, 1815-1820.*
Title: Effectiveness of massage therapy for subacute low-back pain: a randomized controlled trial.
Authors: Preyde, M. (2000).
Conclusions: People with Subacute low back pain were put into 4 groups. The groups were comprehensive massage therapy, soft tissue manipulation only, exercise with posture education, and a placebo group with a sham laser therapy. After 1 month 63% of the comprehensive massage therapy group reported no pain compared to 27% of the soft tissue manipulation group, 14% of the exercise group and 0% of the placebo group.

60. Web link:
http://www.ncbi.nlm.nih.gov/pubmed/11322842
Journal: *Arch Intern Med. 2001 Apr 23;161(8):1081-8.*
Title: Randomized trial comparing traditional Chinese medical acupuncture, therapeutic massage, and self-care education for chronic low back pain.

Authors: Cherkin DC, Eisenberg D, Sherman KJ, Barlow W, Kaptchuk TJ, Street J, Deyo RA.
Conclusions: 262 patients aged 20 to 70 years who had persistent back pain to receive Traditional Chinese Medical acupuncture , therapeutic massage , or self-care educational materials . Up to 10 massage or acupuncture visits were permitted over 10 weeks. At 10 weeks, massage was superior to self-care on the symptom scale. Massage was also superior to acupuncture. After 1 year, massage was not better than self-care but was better than acupuncture. The massage group used the least medications and had the lowest costs of subsequent care.

61. Web link:
http://www.ncbi.nlm.nih.gov/pubmed/7855683
Journal: *Spine, 19*, 2571-2577.
Title: A prospective randomized three-week trial of spinal manipulation, transcutaneous muscle stimulation, massage and corset in the treatment of subacute low back pain.
Authors: Pope, M. H., Phillips, R. B., Haugh, L. D., Hsieh, C. Y., MacDonald, L., and Haldeman, S. (1994).
Conclusions: A randomized study of chiropractic, massage, corset and transcutaneous muscle stimulation (TMS) was conducted in patients with low back pain. Patients were enrolled for a period of 3 weeks and were evaluated once a week by questionnaires, visual analog scale, range of motion, maximum voluntary extension effort, straight leg raising and a fatigue test. After 3 weeks, the chiropractic group scored the greatest

improvements in flexion and pain while the massage group had the best extension effort and fatigue time, and the TMS group the best extension.

62. Web link:
http://nccam.nih.gov/research/results/spotlight/070411.htm
Journal: *Annals of Internal Medicine.* 2011;155(1):1–9.
Title: Massage Therapy Holds Promise for Low-Back Pain
Authors: Cherkin DC, Sherman KJ, Kahn J, et al
Conclusions: 400 patients were randomly assigned to a structural massage group, relaxation massage group, or a usual care group. The usual care group included medications, physical therapy and back exercises. The structural massage group received neuromuscular and musculoskeletal massage and the relaxation massage was Swedish massage. Each massage participant received a 1 hour massage once a week for 10 weeks. The patients were measured by amount of medications, symptoms, and ability to perform activities at 10 weeks, 6 months, and 1 year. Both massage groups showed significant increases in reduction of symptoms and daily functions. At 6 months, the massage groups still showed some improvement, but at 1 year all three groups were the same. This study shows that massage can be helpful in reducing back pain.

Lymph Node Dissection Surgery

63. Web link:
http://web.me.com/touchmaster/nurture/Clinical_Trials.html
Journal: *Cancer Nurs., 27,* 25-33.
Title: Postoperative arm massage: a support for women with lymph node dissection
Authors: Forchuk, C., Baruth, P., Prendergast, M., Holliday, R., Bareham, R., Brimner, S., Schulz, V., Chan, Y.C., Yammine, N. (2004).
Conclusions: Following lymph node dissection surgery, the participant's significant other was taught to perform arm massage as a postoperative support measure. Participants reported a reduction in pain in the immediate postoperative period and better shoulder function.

Migraines

64. Web link: http://www.mendeley.com/research/a-randomized-controlled-trial-of-massage-therapy-as-a-treatment-for-migraine/
Journal: *Annual Behavior and Medicine, 32,* 50-59.
Title- A randomized, controlled trial of massage therapy as a treatment for migraine.
Authors: Lawler, S. & Cameron, L. (2006)
Conclusions: 47 migraine sufferers were randomly divided into 2 groups: massage or control group. All participants completed daily assessments on migraine

experiences and sleep patterns for 13 weeks, Between weeks 5 to 10 the massage group received a weekly massage. Before and after each massage session the participants were assessed on state anxiety, heart rates, and salivary cortisol. Then on weeks 4, 10, and 13 their perceived stress and coping efficacy were assessed. The massage group showed significant improvements during the massage sessions and even the 3 weeks following. During the massage sessions the participants had decreases in state anxiety, heart rate, and cortisol.

Multiple Sclerosis

65. Web link:
http://msj.sagepub.com/content/9/4/356.abstract
Journal: *Multiple Sclerosis, 9*, 356-361.
Title: Reflexology treatment relieves symptoms of multiple sclerosis
Authors: Siev-Ner, I., Gamus, D., Lerner-Geva, L., & Achiron, A. (2003).
Conclusions: 71 people suffering from MS were randomly placed into 2 groups; one group was a control group that received non-specific massage on their calves and the second group that received very specific Reflexology on their feet and calves for 11 weeks. The Reflexology group received pressure on specific points on their feet and calves. The Reflexology group showed significant improvements in parathesias, urinary symptoms, and spasticity even on their 3 month follow-up. Muscle strength improved slightly in both groups.

Nausea

66. Web link:
http://www.ncbi.nlm.nih.gov/pubmed/17309378
Journal: *Journal of Alternative Complementary Medicine. 2007 Jan-Feb;13(1):53-7.*
Title: Massage relieves nausea in women with breast cancer who are undergoing chemotherapy.
Authors: Billhult A, Bergbom I, Stener-Victorin E.
Conclusions: Thirty-nine women, average age of 52 years old, with breast cancer undergoing chemotherapy were enrolled. The patients were randomly assigned to a massage therapy group that received 20 minutes of massage for 5 visits or a control group that just got five 20-minute visits. All patients recorded nausea and anxiety on the Visual Analogue Scale before and after each session. Massage treatment significantly reduced nausea compared with control treatment when improvement was measured as a percentage of the five treatment periods. Differences in anxiety and depression between the two treatment regimes could not be statistically demonstrated. This study complements previous studies on the effect of massage and supports the conclusion that massage reduces nausea in these patients.

67. Web link: http://www.news-medical.net/news/20100417/
Journal: *News Medical, April 17, 2010*
Title: Touch, massage can reduce stress/anxiety, pain,

fatigue, depression and nausea in cancer patients
Author: William Collinge, Ph.D.
Conclusions: The National Cancer Institute sponsored a recent research study which has revealed that touch and massage, routinely administered by family members significantly reduces the effects of cancer and the side-effects from its treatment while providing comfort and improvement in the quality of life. During the study, family caregivers learned touch and massage techniques from an instructional DVD. "The magnitude of the impact of family members was unexpected. Our research found significant reductions of pain, anxiety, fatigue, depression and nausea when massage was routinely administered at home by family and caregivers," states lead researcher William Collinge, Ph.D. The study found massage by family members reduced stress/anxiety (44% reduction), pain (34%), fatigue (32%), depression (31%), and nausea (29%).

68. Web link: http://www.mendeley.com/research/tactile-massage-severe-nausea-vomiting-during-pregnancywomens-experiences/
Journal: *Scandinavian Journal of Caring Sciences (2006)*
Volume: 20, Issue: 2, Pages: 169-176
Title: Tactile massage and severe nausea and vomiting during pregnancy - women's experiences.
Authors: V Newman, J T Fullerton, P O Anderson
Conclusions: 10 women suffering from severe nausea and vomiting during pregnancy were given a tactile massage on 3 different occasions. After the third session

each woman was interviewed about their experience in relaxation and re-gaining control over their bodies. Each of the women suggested that the tactile massage did relaxher body and allow her to re-gain control over her body.

Nervous System

69. Web link:
http://www.ncbi.nlm.nih.gov/pubmed/19283590
Journal: *International Journal of Neuroscience. 2009;119(5):630-8.*
Title- Moderate pressure massage elicits a parasympathetic nervous system response.
Authors: Diego MA, Field T.
Conclusions: Twenty healthy adults were randomly assigned to a moderate pressure or a light pressure massage therapy group. EKGs were recorded during a 3-min baseline, during the 15-min massage period, and during a 3-min post massage period. The participants who received the moderate pressure massage exhibited a parasympathetic nervous system response characterized by an increase in High Frequency, suggesting increased vagal efferent nerve activity and a decrease in the Low Frequency/High Frequency ratio, suggesting a shift from sympathetic to parasympathetic activity that peaked during the first half of the massage period. On the other hand, those who received the light pressure massage exhibited a sympathetic nervous system response characterized by decreased High

Frequency and increased Low Frequency/High Frequency. The higher the pressure of massage, the higher the nerve activity was throughout the body.

Neuropathy

70. Web link:
http://www.sciencedirect.com/science/article/pii/S105532900600197X
Journal: *Journal of the Association of Nurses in AIDS care*
Volume 17, Issue 5, September-October 2006, Pages 15-22
Title: Effects of Ice Massage on Neuropathic Pain in Persons With AIDS
Authors: Kristin Kane Ownby PhD, RN, ACRN, AOCN, CHPN
Conclusions: 33 patients suffering from neuropathic pain from AIDS were used in this pilot study. Three treatments were used: ice massage, towel massage, and presence. The purpose of this study was to see if ice massage would affect the pain intensity and improve sleep quality. While the results of the study were negative, there was a decrease in pain intensity over time with the ice massage and towel massage. This would warrant further studies to learn more about the affects massage could have on neuropathies.

Osgood-Schlatter Disease

71. Web link:
http://emedicine.medscape.com/article/827380-overview
Journal: *Medscape reference (online), May 5, 2010*
Title: Osgood-Schlatter Disease in Emergency Medicine
Authors: Andrew K Chang, MD; Chief Editor: Rick Kulkarni, MD
Conclusions: Among adolescents, Osgood-Schlatter's Disease is one of the most common causes of knee pain. According to one Finnish study, Osgood-Schlatter's Disease occurs in about 13% of athletes and is particularly prevalent among teenage boys. It is a painful affliction of the knees which can last months or even years. Since bone growth is faster than soft tissue growth, muscle tendons can become tight across the joint resulting in edema and loss of flexibility. Corticosteroids are not recommended. The most effective therapy involves quadriceps and hamstring stretching exercises and extending the hip for a complete stretch of the extensor mechanism to reduce tension on the tibial tubercle.

Osteoarthritis

72. Web link:
http://www.ncbi.nlm.nih.gov/pubmed/17159021
Journal: *Arch Intern Med. 2006 Dec 11-25;166(22):2533-8.*

Title: Massage therapy for osteoarthritis of the knee: a randomized controlled trial.
Authors: Perlman AI, Sabina A, Williams AL, Njike VY, Katz DL.
Source: Institute for Complementary and Alternative Medicine, University of Medicine and Dentistry of New Jersey, School of Health Realted Profession, Newark, NJ 07107-1709, USA. a.perlman@umdnj.edu
Conclusions: Sixty-eight adults with osteoarthritis (OA) of the knee were assigned either to a control group or for twice weekly sessions of Swedish massage for 4 weeks, then once weekly for four weeks. Primary outcomes were measured via changes in the Western Ontario and McMaster Universities Osteoarthritis Index (WOMAC) pain and functional scores and the visual analog scale of pain assessment. Those receiving massage demonstrated a significant reduction in pain and stiffness and the time it took to walk 50 feet and a significant increase in range of movement. Findings indicate that massage therapy is an effective treatment for OA of the knee.

73. Web link: *http://www.massage-research.com/blog/?p=781*
Journal: *2009 Journal of Geriatric Physical Therapy 32 (3), pp. 111-116*
Title: Can stimulating massage improve joint repositioning error in patients with knee osteoarthritis?
Authors: Lund, H., Henriksen, M., Bartels, E.M., Danneskiold-Samsøe, B., Bliddal, H.

Conclusions: Nineteen (19) patients with osteoarthritis of the knee who suffered from joint repositioning error of the knee were treated with 10 minutes of massage to the quadriceps femoris, sartorious, gracilus, and hamstrings muscles on the affected leg. The mean age of these patients was 73.1 years. After one massage therapy session, there was no significant change in their joint repositioning error. [This is asking a lot from one 10 minute massage session!]

Oxytocin Levels

74. Web link:
http://www.sciencedirect.com/science/article/pii/0165183895000567
Journal: *Journal of the Autonomic Nervous System, 56, 26-30.*
Title: Massage-like stroking of the abdomen lowers blood pressure in anesthetized rats: influence of oxytocin
Authors: Kurosawa, M., Lundeberg, T., Agren, G., Lund, I., and Uvnas-Moberg, K. (1995)
Conclusions: Massage-like stroking for one minute of the ventral area of the abdomen anaesthetized rats raised oxytocin levels and lowered their blood pressure, and more so than if the lateral sides of the abdomen were massaged. Blood pressure returned to its initial level one minute after stroking stopped. [Important information when massaging hypertensive rats]

Pain

75. Web link:
http://top25.sciencedirect.com/subject/nursing-and-health-professions/19/journal/complementary-therapies-in-clinical-practice/17443881/archive/27
Journal: *Complementary Therapies in Clinical Practice, 16*, 92-95.
Title: Effect of massage therapy on pain, anxiety, and tension in cardiac surgical patients: a pilot study.
Authors: Cutshall, S.M., Wentworth, L.J., Engen, D., Sundt, T.M., Kely, R.F., & Bauer, B.A. (2010).
Conclusions: Two to five days after undergoing cardiovascular surgical procedures, patients were given a 20 minute session of massage therapy. Compared to those who received standard care, those patients receiving massage exhibited significant decreases in pain, anxiety, and tension.

76. Web link:
http://top25.sciencedirect.com/subject/nursing-and-health-professions/19/journal/journal-of-bodywork-and-movement-therapies/13608592/archive/13
Journal: *Journal of Bodywork and Movement Therapy, 11*, 141-145.
Title: Lower back pain and sleep disturbance are reduced following massage therapy.

Authors: Field, T., Hernandez-Reif, M., Diego, M., & Fraser, M. (2007)
Conclusions: Thirty adults with a mean age of 41 years who had lower back pain for at least six months were treated with massage therapy twice weekly for five (5) weeks. Sessions were 30 minutes long. Their results were contrasted with a control group who used progressive muscle relaxation therapy which involved tensing and relaxing large muscle groups. Those in the massage group reported having less depressed mood, less anxiety, and less pain. Their results were better than for those in the relaxation group.

77. Web link:
http://www.ncbi.nlm.nih.gov/pubmed/14665792
Journal: *Psychother Psychosom., 73,* 17-24.
Title: A randomized clinical trial of the treatment effects of massage compared to relaxation tape recordings on diffuse long-term pain.
Authors: Hasson, D., Arnetz, B., Jelveus, L., & Edelstam, B. (2004)
Conclusions: The purpose of this study was to determine if, among those with long term musculoskeletal pain, massage were more effective than listening to relaxation tapes at significantly improving patients' self-rated health, levels of muscle pain, and mental energy. 129 patients were divided into two groups, and improvements in these areas were only observed in the massage group.

78. Web link: *http://www.nammt.co.uk/research.php*
Journal: *Journal of Bodywork & Movement Therapies, 12, 146-150.*
Title: Massage therapy reduces pain in pregnant women, alleviates prenatal depression in both parents and improves their relationships.
Authors: Field, T., Figueiredo, B., Hernandez-Reif, M., Diego, M., Deeds, O. & Ascencio, A. (2008).
Conclusions: Forty-seven depressed and pregnant women were either assigned to a control group or were massaged by their partners twice a week from 20 weeks of pregnancy until their delivery. Those receiving the massages reported less back pain, leg pain, depression, anger, and anxiety than those in the control group. Also, the partners giving the massages reported less anger, anxiety, and depression. Moreover those involved in the massage group reported that their relationships improved. [Massage works! Who knew?]

79. Web link:
http://www.sciencedirect.com/science/article/pii/S1353611799904298
Journal: *Complementary Therapies in Nursing & Midwifery, 6, 25-32.*
Title: Effect of cutaneous stimulation on pain reduction in emergency department patients.
Authors: Kubsch, S.M., Neveau, T., & Vandertie, K. (2000).

Conclusions: Fifty emergency room patients were treated with massage (tactile stimulation) to relieve pain. Thereafter the patients reported less pain, and objective findings showed that heart rate and blood pressure dropped.

80. Web link: *http://www6.miami.edu/touch-research/Massage.html*
Journal: *Journal of Pediatric Psychology, 34, 1096-1096.*
Title: A randomized controlled trial of massage therapy in children with sickle cell disease.
Authors: Lemanek, K.L., Ranalli, M., Lukens, C. (2009).
Conclusions: Children were assigned at random either to a control group or to be massaged nightly by their parents. Those receiving massage showed less pain, depression and anxiety and were able to function at a higher level.

81. Web link:
http://www.sciencedirect.com/science/article/pii/0304395984908078
Journal: *Pain, 20, 13-23.*
Title: Long-term results of vibratory stimulation as a pain relieving measure for chronic pain.
Authors: Lundeberg, T. (1984).
Conclusions: Two hundred sixty-seven (267) patients were treated with vibratory stimulation for 18 months to relieve chronic musculoskeletal and neurogenic pain.

More than half of those treated - 59% - reported that their pain was reduced by more than 50%. Of those who reported significant pain relief (the 59%), after 12 months of home treatment with a vibratory massage stimulator, 72% increased their social activity and more than 50% reduced their intake of pain killing drugs.

82. Web link: *http://www.mendeley.com/research/effect-of-vibratory-stimulation-on-experimental-and-clinical-pain/*
Journal: Scandinavian Journal of Rehabilitation Medicine, 20, 149-159.
Title: Effect of vibratory stimulation on experimental and clinical pain.
Authors: Lundeberg, T., Abrahamsson, P., Bondesson, L., & Haker, E. (1987).
Conclusions: Vibratory stimulation was performed on the left and right extensor carpi radialis longus muscles of 16 healthy patients and 18 patients who suffered from chronic epicondylitis of the right elbow. Thereafter there was no difference in pain thresholds among the healthy patients; but among those suffering epicondylitis, the pain thresholds increased by 120% to 230%. Twelve of the epicondylitis patients reported pain relief for a span of 1 to 7 hours.

83. Web link: *http://www.biomedcentral.com/1472-6882/6/20*
Journal: *BMC Complementary and Alternative Medicine* 2006, 6:20
Title: Vibratory stimulation increases the electro-cutaneous sensory detection and pain thresholds in women but not in men
Authors: Dahlin, Lund, Lundeberg, Molander
Conclusions: Although this study confirmed that electro-vibratory stimulation is useful for treating pain, the beneficial effects were surprisingly limited only to women.

84. Web link:
http://www.mendeley.com/research/vibratory-stimulation-compared-to-placebo-in-alleviation-of-pain/
Journal: *Scandinavian Journal of Rehabilitation Medicine, 19, 153-158.*
Title: Vibratory stimulation compared to placebo in alleviation of pain.
Authors: Lundeberg, T., Abrahamsson, P., & Haker, E. (1987).
Conclusions: In a double-blind crossover trial using a vibrator and a "placebo unit" vibratory stimulator on 72 patients to study the placebo effect with chronic pain syndromes, it was determined that 48% of the patients reported pain relief using the real vibrator and 34% reported relief using the placebo vibrator.

85. Web links: *http://www.21stcenturymed.org/fhti-hwb6-final.pdf*
Journal: *Australian Journal of Advanced Nursing, 14, 21-26.*
Title: Expanding the nursing repertoire: The effect of massage on post-operative pain.
Authors: Nixon, M., Teschendorff, J., Finney, J., & Karnilowicz, W. (1997).
Conclusions: Nineteen patients with post-operative pain were treated with massage and compared to a control group of twenty people. Those massaged reported a significant reduction in pain for 24 hours after their massage.

86. Web link: *http://www.journalacs.org/article/S1072-7515(03)00992-X/fulltext*
Journal: *Journal of the American College of Surgeons, 197, 1037-1046.*
Title: Massage as adjuvant therapy in the management of acute postoperative pain: a preliminary study in men.
Authors: Piotrowski, M.M., Paterson, C., Mitchinson, A., Kim, H.M., Kirsh, M., Hinshaw, D.B. (2003).
Conclusions: After major operations, 202 patients were treated randomly with either massage, focused attention, or routine care to assess the impact of each intervention on pain relief. Perceived amount of post-op pain declined significantly in those treated with massage; however, they still took the same amount of opioid analgesics.

87. Web link: *http://www.mendeley.com/research/trial-effectiveness-soft-tissue-massage-treatment-shoulder-pain/*
Journal: *The Australian Journal of Physiotherapy, 49,* 183-188.
Title: A trial into the effectiveness of soft tissue massage in the treatment of shoulder pain.
Authors: Van den Dolder, P.A., & Roberts, D.L. (2003).
Conclusions: In a single blinded, randomized controlled study of 29 patients with shoulder pain, soft tissue massage significantly improved range of motion, level of pain, and function.

88. Web link: *http://www.positivehealth.com/research/walach-and-co-workers*
Journal: *Journal of Alternative and Complementary Medicine, 9, 837-846.*
Title: Efficacy of massage therapy in chronic pain: A pragmatic randomized trial.
Authors: Walach, H., Guthlin, C., & Konig, M. (2003).
Conclusions: This study compared standard medical care (SMC) to massage for patients with chronic pain of the head, neck, back, shoulders, and limbs. Ten patients were given SMC, and nineteen were treated with massage. Both groups experienced pain relief and decreased depression and anxiety, but only in the massage group did the reduction in pain, depression, and anxiety last until the follow up at three months.

89. Web link:
http://www.ncbi.nlm.nih.gov/pubmed/15297952
Journal: *Pain Management Nursing, 5, 59-65.*
Title: Foot and hand massage as an intervention for postoperative pain.
Authors: Wang, H.L., & Keck, J.F. (2004).
Conclusions: Postoperative patients in pain were given foot and hand massages for 20 minutes (five minutes per extremity). They reported less pain thereafter, and the objective findings were reduced heart and respiratory rates.

90. Web link:
http://www.medscape.com/viewarticle/559775_4
Journal: *Medscape*
Title: Effectiveness of Massage Therapy for Chronic, Non-malignant Pain: A Review: Discussion
Authors: Jennie C.I. Tsao, Pediatric Pain Program, Department of Pediatrics, David Geffen School of Medicine at UCLA, USA
Conclusions: According to a Cochrane review, there is strong evidence that massage is effective in treating lower back pain. There is also strong evidence that massage is effective at relieving shoulder pain. There was less evidence of pain relief for the following ailments, in descending order of effectiveness: headache pain, fibromyalgia, mixed chronic pain, neck pain and Carpal Tunnel Syndrome. The study also discusses

three main hypotheses for why massage is effective at relieving pain: gate theory, the serotonin hypothesis, and the restorative sleep hypothesis.

Parkinson's Disease

91. Web link:
http://www.sciencedirect.com/science/article/pii/S1360859202902822
Journal: *Journal of Bodywork and Movement Therapies, 6,* 177-182.
Title: Parkinson's disease symptoms are reduced by massage therapy and progressive muscle exercises.
Authors: Hernandez-Reif, M., Field, T., Largie, S., Cullen, C., Beutler, J., Sanders, C., Weiner, W., Rodriguez-Bateman, D., Zelaya, L., Schanberg, S. & Kuhn, C. (2002).
Conclusions: Sixteen Parkinson's patients were given massage for 30 minutes twice a week for five weeks or else given sessions of progressive muscle relaxation. Those who received massage reported that they had improved their daily functioning and also slept better. Moreover, their physicians reported that the massage patients had improved in daily living activities.

Patellafemoral Pain Syndrome - PFPS (Runner's Knee)

92. Web link:
http://www2.cochrane.org/reviews/en/ab003375.html
Journal: *Cochrane Database of Systematic Reviews 2001, Issue 4. Art. No.: CD003375. DOI: 10.1002/14651858.CD003375*
Title: Therapeutic ultrasound for treating patellofemoral pain syndrome
Authors: Brosseau L, Casimiro L, Welch V, Milne S, Shea B, Judd M, Wells GA, Tugwell P.
Conclusions: The Cochrane database search retrieved 85 articles on treatment of Patellafemoral pain syndrome of which only one was appropriate for review. This study was focused on the efficacy of treating this syndrome with Ultrasound in addition to ice massage which is the standard mode of care. There were 53 participants in the study. All patients underwent an exercise protocol. Four of the thirteen patients (31%) treated with ice massage alone reported less patellafemoral pain and/or quadriceps/hamstring strengthening compared with 6 of 16 (46%) who received both ultrasound and ice massage. Clearly the ice massage was of some benefit, but the improvement with ultrasound was only 15% more, not enough to meet the international standard of 20% for clinically important improvements in the treatment of osteoarthritis.

93. Web link:
http://www.ncbi.nlm.nih.gov/pubmed/21589717
Journal: *Int J Ther Massage Bodywork. 2008 Dec 15;1(2):11-21.*
Title: Massage therapy protocol for post-anterior cruciate ligament reconstruction patellofemoral pain syndrome (PFPS): a case report.
Author: J. Zalta
Conclusions: In this case study, one patient with PFPS was treated with various massage techniques including
- neuromuscular therapy with trigger point release
- myofascial release
- lymphatic drainage
- cross-fiber friction
- and muscle energy techniques.

To chart changes in range of motion in the knee and patellafemoral function, the doctor used orthopedic physical assessment tests including
- Pre- and post-massage heel-height difference, measuring degree of hamstring flexion contracture.
- Anthropometric measurements tracking effusion and atrophy pre- and post surgery
- pre- and post-massage pain level (PL) on a scale of 1 to 10 for each session

These tests documented a decrease in hamstring flexion contracture, a decrease in lateral tracking of the patella, and a decrease in pain level – all indicating that massage therapies are effective modalities for the treatment of PFPS.

Perineal Massage

94. Web link:
http://www.mendeley.com/research/prenatal-perineal-massage-preventing-lacerations-during-delivery/
Journal: *JOGNN - Journal of Obstetric, Gynecologic, & Neonatal Nursing, 29, 474-479.*
Title: Prenatal perineal massage: preventing lacerations during delivery.
Authors: Davidson, K., Jacoby, S., & Brown, M.S. (2000).
Conclusions: In a study of 368 expectant women, prenatal perineal massage was the one factor – other than frequency of births – which determined favorably how serious a mother's perineum tore during childbirth.

95. Web link:
http://www.oxfordradcliffe.nhs.uk/forpatients/090427patientinfoleaflets/090924perinealmassage.pdf
Journal: *British Journal of Obstetrics & Gynaecology, 108, 499-504.*
Title: Women's views on the practice of prenatal perineal massage.
Authors: Labrecque, M., Eason, E., & Marcoux, S. (2001).
Conclusions: 763 pregnant women received perineal massage and reported the following:
   1. the massage had a positive effect on their preparation for birth

2. the more their husbands participated the better effect it had on their relationships
3. most women said they would recommend perineal massage to other pregnant women and would do it if pregnant again

Peripheral Neuropathy

96. Web link:
http://gateway.nlm.nih.gov/MeetingAbstracts/ma?f=102231174.html
Journal: *Int Conf AIDS. 1998; 12: 849 (abstract no. 42376).*
Title: Massage therapy for the treatment of painful peripheral neuropathy in HIV+ individuals.
Authors: Acosta AM, Chan RS, Jacobs J; International Conference on AIDS.
Conclusions: Massage therapy was used to treat peripheral neuropathy in five non-diabetic patients with HIV and two diabetic patients with HIV who previously had little or no positive response to pharmacologic therapy. It significantly decreased foot pain in all five of the non-diabetic patients, but the diabetic patients showed no improvement.

Physicians' Perspectives

97. Web link: *http://www6.miami.edu/touch-research/Massage.html*
Journal: *Canadian Family Physician, 44, 1018-1040.*
Title: Physicians' perspectives on massage therapy.
Authors: Verhoef, M.J., & Page, S.A. (1998).
Conclusions: 162 Canadian family physicians were questioned about massage therapy; and 68% said they had minimal or no knowledge about it. Of those 32% who indicated some knowledge about massage, 83% said it was a useful adjunct to their practice of medicine; 72% said their patients were asking more and more for massage therapy; and 71% had referred to a massage therapist. Those who referred to massage therapists had more positive views about massage and more knowledge about massage therapy. Half of the physicians questioned supported laws to regulate massage therapy.

Physiological Responses to Massage

98. Web link:
http://onlinelibrary.wiley.com/doi/10.1046/j.1365-2648.2002.02103.x/full
Journal: *Journal of Advanced Nursing, 37, 364-371.*
Title: The short-term effects of myofascial trigger point massage therapy on cardiac autonomic tone in healthy subjects.

Authors: Delaney, J.P., Leong, K.S., Watkins, A., & Brodie, D. (2002).
Conclusions: Thirty healthy subjects were treated with myofascial trigger point massage to the head, neck, and shoulders. Their blood pressure was taken before and after the sessions, and they rated their levels of muscle tension and emotional states. After massage their heart rates dropped, as did their systolic and diastolic blood pressures. They also reported improvements in their levels of muscle tension and emotional states.

99. Web link:
http://www.ingentaconnect.com/content/apl/gnes/2004/00000114/00000001/art00003
Journal: *International Journal of Neuroscience, 114, 31-44.*
Title: Massage therapy of moderate and light pressure and vibrator effects on EEG and heart rate.
Authors: Diego, M.A., Field, T., Sanders, C., & Hernandez-Reif, M. (2004).
Conclusions: 36 healthy adults were treated with three types of massage and randomly assigned to three groups: light massage, moderate massage, and vibratory stimulation. Although all groups reported a decrease in anxiety, those receiving the moderate pressure experienced the greatest reduction in stress, heart rate, and EEG changes – the latter showing a decrease in beta and alpha wave activity and an increase in delta wave activity, indicative of relaxation. The light massage and vibratory groups showed increased levels of arousal as indicated by increased heart rates and beta levels.

The vibratory group also showed increased levels of alpha and theta wave activity.

Plantar Fasciitis

100. Web link:
http://www.aafp.org/afp/2001/0201/p467.html
Journal: *Am Fam Physician.* 2001 Feb 1;63(3):467-475.
Title: Treatment of Plantar Fasciitis
Authors: CRAIG C. YOUNG, M.D., DARIN S. RUTHERFORD, M.D., MARK W. NIEDFELDT, M.D.,
Conclusions: This article in the journal *American Family Physician* surveys the various treatments for plantar fasciitis and reports that stretching is considered the most effective, as it can correct risk factors such as weakness of the foot muscles and tightness of the gastrocnemius muscles. The authors recommend that, before getting out of bed in the morning, patients do self cross-fiber friction massage above the plantar fascia and stretch with a towel. They also recommend the following stretching techniques:
- wall stretching
- curb or stair stretches
- using a slant board
- placing a 2"x 4" piece of wood in workplaces where the patient stands for long periods of time so they patient can stretch his/her calf muscles
- rolling the foot over a tennis ball or a 15 oz. can

Posttraumatic Stress

101. Web link:
http://www.massagetherapycanada.com/content/view/1281/38/
Journal: *Journal of Applied Developmental Psychology, 17, 37-50.*
Title: Alleviating posttraumatic stress in children following Hurricane Andrew.
Authors: Field, T., Seligman, S., Scafidi, F., & Schanberg, S. (1996).
Conclusions: Following Hurricane Andrew, sixty students from grades 1-5 with behavior problems in the classroom who exhibited Posttraumatic Stress Disorder by their scores on the PTSD Index were randomly assigned to two groups: one received massage, the other watched videos. Those receiving massage reported they were happier and less anxious, and their saliva showed reduced levels of cortisol after massage than the levels exhibited by the video group. Those massaged also had lower scores for depression and anxiety and were more relaxed.

Pregnancy

102. Web link: *http://www6.miami.edu/touch-research/AdultMassage.html*
Journal: *Journal of Psychosomatic Obstetrics & Gynecology, 20, 31-38.*
Title: Pregnant women benefit from massage therapy.
Authors: Field, T., Hernandez-Reif, M., Hart, S., Theakston, H., Schanberg, S., Kuhn, C. & Burman, I. (1999).
Conclusions: For five weeks, 26 pregnant women were either massaged twice a week for 20 minutes or assigned to a relaxation group. Although women from each group reported less leg pain after the first and last sessions, after the last session only the women in the massage group reported:
- reduced anxiety
- improved mood
- less back pain
- better sleep
- low levels of norepinephrine (urinary stress hormone levels)
- fewer complications during labor
- fewer premature births
- fewer postnatal complications

103. Web link:
http://www.ingentaconnect.com/content/apl/spri/2001/00 000019/00000001/art00012
Journal: *Scandinavian Journal of Primary Health Care, 19, 43-47.*
Title: Acupressure treatment of morning sickness in pregnancy. A randomized, double-blind, placebo-controlled study.
Authors: Norheim, A.J., Pederson, E.J., Fonnebo, V., & Berge, L. (2001).
Conclusions: 97 pregnant women were studied during their 8th to 12th weeks of gestation to determine if acupressure could alleviate symptoms of morning sickness. Of those women massaged, 71% reported less intense nausea and vomiting and for reduced duration.

104. Web link:
http://preventdisease.com/news/articles/acupressure_ea se_morning_sickness.shtml
Journal: *The Journal of Reproductive Medicine, 46, 835-839.*
Title: Effect of acupressure on nausea and vomiting during pregnancy. A randomized, placebo-controlled, pilot study.
Authors: Werntoft, E., & Dykes, A.K. (2001).
Conclusions: Pregnant women experiencing morning sickness were divided into two groups. A pressure band with a button was applied to acupuncture point Pericardium 6 (P6) in one group and to a placebo point

in another group. Those in the P6 group reported continuing relief from nausea symptoms through the 14th day of the study. Those in the placebo group experienced relief only through the 6th day.

105. Web link: *http://www6.miami.edu/touch-research/InfantMassage.html*
Journal: *Infant Behavior and Development, 29, 54-58.*
Title: Newborns of depressed mothers who received moderate versus light pressure massage during pregnancy.
Authors: Field, T., Hernandez-Reif, M., & Diego, M. (2006).
Conclusions: This study was of sixty-four babies, born of two groups of depressed pregnant women who were massaged during their 5th through 8th month of pregnancy. One group of mothers was massaged with light stimulation; the other with moderate stimulation. After childbirth, their newborn babies (average age of 6.8 days) were examined for 15 minutes and for their performance on the Brazelton Neonatal Behavior Assessment Scale. Those infants of mothers who received moderate pressure massage received better scores on the Brazelton Scale on depression, excitability, motor, and orientation clusters and were observed to spend more time smiling and vocalizing.

106. Web link:
http://www.ncbi.nlm.nih.gov/pmc/articles/PMC2262938/
Journal: *Infant Behav Dev. 2008 January; 31(1): 149–152.*
Title: Temperature Increases in Preterm Infants During Massage Therapy
Authors: Miguel A. Diego, Tiffany Field, and Maria Hernandez-Reif
Conclusions: Preterm babies are at risk for hypothermia (low body temperature) and are kept in isolettes with the portholes closed to preserve their body heat. There has been much research which shows that neonatal massage is highly beneficial. Preterm newborns receiving massage are hospitalized 3-6 days less than those preterms not receiving massage. Also, they gain 21-47% more weight than their non-massaged counterparts. As a result, massage therapy is practiced in 38% of the neonatal Intensive Care Units around the country. (Field, Hernandez-Reif & Diego, 2006). This study was performed to determine if massage to preterm babies (which necessitated opening the portholes) would lower their body temperatures unduly. In this study 72 preterm infants were assigned either to a massage group or to a control group. The massage group received three 15 minute sessions a day, comprising of

1. 5 minutes of massage with moderate pressure to the neck, shoulders, along the spine and back, waist, and arms and legs
2. 5 minutes of moving the limbs
3. A repeat of step 1.

Those in the massage group actually exhibited increased temperatures over those in the control group, confirming that massaged pre-term infants are not at risk for increased temperature loss.

107. Web link:
http://www.ncbi.nlm.nih.gov/pubmed/17138258
Journal: *Infant Behav Dev. 2006 Jan;29(1):24-31. Epub 2005 Oct 28.*
Title: Prenatal, perinatal and neonatal stimulation: a survey of neonatal nurseries.
Authors: Field T, Hernandez-Reif M, Feijo L, Freedman J.
Conclusions: 82 staff members from Neonatal Intensive care Units (NICU's) were surveyed to discover what types of stimulation pregnant mothers and babies received. These were the results:
- breastfeeding in the NICU (100%).
- kangaroo care (98%);
- non-nutritive sucking during tube feedings in the NICU (96%);
- containment (swaddling and surrounded by blanket rolls) in the NICU (86%);
- rocking in the NICU (85%);

- skin-to-skin following birth in the delivery room (83% of hospitals);
- music in the NICU (72%);
- preterm infant massage in the NICU (38%).
- labor massage (30%);
- the Doula (assistant who comforts during labor and delivery) (30%)
- waterbeds in the NICU (23%); and
- pregnancy massage (19%);

108. Web link:
http://www.ncbi.nlm.nih.gov/pubmed/18780582
Journal: *Alternative Therapies in Health and Medicine, 14, 28-34.*
Title: Pregnancy and Labor Alternative Therapy Research.
Authors: Field, T. (2008)
Conclusions: Massage and other alternative therapies are effective at reducing pregnancy related depression, nausea, premature births, leg and back pain, pain during childbirth, and concomitantly reduced need for medication.

Premature births

109. Web link:
http://informahealthcare.com/doi/abs/10.1080/00207450701239327?journalCode=nes
Journal: *International Journal of Neuroscience, 118, 277-289.*
Title: Prematurity and Potential Predictors.
Authors: Field, T. Diego, M., & Hernandez-Reif, M. (2008).
Conclusions: Several factors contribute to premature birth, and these are examined in this article. Among them are high levels of cortisol, and the study identifies massage therapy as way to reduce cortisol levels in pregnancy and thus to reduce the incidence of premature birth.

110. Web link:
http://www.mendeley.com/research/massage-therapy-improves-neurodevelopment-outcome-years-corrected-age-low-birth-weight-infants-6/
Journal: *Early Human Development, 86, 7-11.*
Title: Massage therapy improves neurodevelopmental outcome at two years corrected age for very low birth weight infants.
Authors: Procianoy, R.S., Mendes, E.W. & Silveira, R.C. (2010).
Conclusions: Compared to a control group, premature newborns with very low birthweight who had received massage by their mothers scored a bit higher on

Psychomotor Development and Mental Development Indexes.

Premenstrual Syndrome

111. Web link: *http://www6.miami.edu/touch-research/AdultMassage.html*
Journal: *Journal of Psychosomatic Obstetrics & Gynecology, 21, 9-15.*
Title: Premenstrual syndrome symptoms are relieved by massage therapy.
Authors: Hernandez-Reif, M., Martinez, A., Field, T., Quintero, O., & Hart, S. (2000).
Conclusions: Symptoms of premenstrual syndrome are relieved by massage therapy. This conclusion was the result of a study of 24 premenstrual women who were randomly assigned either to a massage or a relaxation therapy group. Following their massages, those in the massage group experienced less
- anxiety
- pain
- depressed mood
- water retention

Preschool Massage

112. Web link:
http://en.wikipedia.org/wiki/Pediatric_massage
Journal: *Early Child Development and Care, 120, 39-44.*
Title: Preschool children's sleep and wake behavior: Effects of massage therapy.
Authors: Field, T., Kilmer, T., Hernandez-Reif, M. & Burman, I. (1996).
Conclusions: For five weeks some preschool children received 20 minute sessions of massage therapy twice a week. Compared to those children in a control group who did not receive massage, by the end of the study the massage group children were observed to have

- better behavior ratings for activity, cooperation, and vocalization
- better behavior ratings from teachers
- less aversion to touch and more extroversion as judged by their parents
- less time needed to fall asleep during naptime

113. Web link:
http://www.tandfonline.com/doi/abs/10.1080/0300443981430105#preview
Journal: *Early Child Development and Care, 143, 59-64.*
Title: Preschoolers' cognitive performance improves following massage.
Authors: Hart, S.; Field, T.; Hernandez-Reif, M.; & Lundy, B. (1998).

Conclusions: Following a 15 minute massage, preschool students exhibited increased scores for abstract reasoning on the Block Design test of the Wechsler Preschool and Primary Scale of Intelligence (WPPSI). Those children who were judged to be high strung and anxious benefited the most from massage.

114. Web link:
http://www.sacredmotherdoula.com/pdfs/Web%20IM%20Research.pdf
Journal: *Pre and Perinatal Psychology Journal, 11, 73-78.*
Title: Oil Versus No Oil Massage
Authors: Field, T., T., Schanberg, S., Davalos, M. & Malphurs, J. (1996).
Conclusions: A comparison study was done massaging infants – with oil and without oil. When massaged with oil, the infants showed less grimacing and clenching of fists (both stress behaviors) and lower levels of cortisol (a stress hormone).

Preterm Infants

115. Web links:
a)http://www.pediatrics.aappublications.org/content/77/5/654

b) *http://www.nichd.nih.gov/cochrane/vickers/vickers.htm*
c) *http://www.sciencedirect.com/science/article/pii/0163638838690041X*

Journal: *Pediatrics, 77, 654-658.*
Title: Tactile/kinesthetic stimulation effects on preterm neonates.
Authors: Field, T., Schanberg, S., Scafidi, F., Bauer, C., Vega-Lahr, N., Garcia, R., Nystrom, J., & Kuhn, C. (1986).
Conclusions: 20 preterm infants with a mean gestational age of 31 weeks and a mean birth weight of 1,280 grams who had spent a mean time of 20 days in NeoNatal Intensive Care Units (NCIU) were given massage and kinesthetic stimulation for three 15 minute periods per day for 10 days. For 5 minutes they were massaged with moderate pressure, for five minutes their limbs were moved, and for five minutes they were massaged again with moderate pressure. Compared to a control group, the infants who were massaged gained an average of 47% more weight per day, were more alert and active, and on the Brazelton scale showed more mature habituation, motor, orientation, and range of state behavior than those neonates not massaged. Their hospital stays averaged six days less at a savings of about $3,000 per child.

116. Web link:
http://www.springerlink.com/content/g8147n832tll3060/
Journal: *Pediatric Nursing, 13, 385-387.*
Title: Massage of preterm newborns to improve growth and development.
Authors: Field, T., Scafidi, F., and Schanberg, S. (1987).
Conclusions: Preterm newborns who received massage therapy persisted for six months in maintaining more weight gain and better performance on development tests than those preterms not massaged.

117. Web link: *http://www.deepdyve.com/lp/mary-ann-liebert/advances-in-touch-new-implications-in-human-development-fFwfMXL0B6*
Journal: *Advances in Touch. Skillman, N. J.*
Title: Massage alters growth and catecholamine production in preterm newborns.
Authors: Field, T. & Schanberg, S. M. (1990).
Conclusions: This study appears in the book, *Advances in Touch*, and documents the progress of 40 preterm infants who received three 15 minute sessions of massage, kinetic exercise, and massage for three consecutive hours for ten days. Compared to a control group receiving the same caloric intake, these infants gained an average of 21% more weight during the ten days. Also, they spent less time sleeping, grimacing, mouthing/yawning, and clenching their fists. This study was repeated by Scafidi, F.A., Field, T.M., Schanberg, S.M., Bauer, C.R., Tucci, K., Roberts, J., Morrow, C., &

Kuhn, C.M. (1990) – "Massage stimulates growth in preterm infants: A replication." *Infant Behavior and Development, 13,* 167-188. Their results confirmed the earlier findings. Also, those infants massaged were discharged from the hospital 5 days earlier than those in the control group.

118. Web link:
http://www.springerlink.com/content/g8147n832tll3060/
Journal: *Journal of Developmental & Behavioral Pediatrics ,14*, 176-180.
Title: Factors that predict which preterm infants benefit most from massage therapy.
Authors: Scafidi, F. A., Field, T., & Schanberg, S. M. (1993).
Conclusions: 70% of pre-term infants who received massage therapy were considered high weight gainers compared to only 40% of infants in the control group who were high weight gainers. Those preterm infants who had experienced obstetric complications benefited the most from massage therapy.

119. Web link:
http://journals.lww.com/jrnldbp/toc/1993/10000
Journal: *Journal of Developmental & Behavioral Pediatrics, 14*, 318-322.
Title: Massage effects on cocaine-exposed preterm neonates.
Authors: Wheeden, A., Scafidi, F. A., Field, T., Ironson, G., Valdeon, C., and Bandstra, E. (1993).

Conclusions: Thirty pre-term infants who had been exposed to cocaine and had a mean gestational period of 30 weeks were divided into two groups. Fifteen served as a control group, and 15 received a combination of massage-kinetic activity-massage for 15 minutes for three hours in a row for ten days. Compared to the control group, those receiving the massage
1. gained on average 28% more weight per day
2. exhibited better motor behaviors on the Brazelton scale at the end of ten days
3. exhibited statistically significant less complications after birth and fewer stress behaviors

120. Web link:

http://snrs.org/publications/SOJNR_articles2/Vol10Num03Art05.html
Journal: *Journal of Music Therapy, 37, 250-268.*
Title: The effect of parent training in music and multimodal stimulation on parent-neonate interactions in the neonatal intensive care unit.
Author: Whipple, J. (2000)
Conclusions: Twenty sets of parents received one hour of instruction in the use of music and massage techniques to treat their premature infants borne with low birth weights. Observations were done of the interactions between parents and children and the infants' stress and non-stress responses. Parents who received the training acted and responded more appropriately to their infants, and the infants exhibited significantly less stress behavior. Also these parents spent significantly more

time in the NCIU than parents of the control group who did not receive such training.

121. Web link: *http://www6.miami.edu/touch-research/InfantMassage.html*
Journal: Current Directions in Psychological Science, 10, 51-54.
Title: Massage therapy facilitates weight gain in preterm infants.
Author: Field, T. (2001).
Conclusions: Premature newborns who received three 15 minute sessions of massage-kinetic activity-massage three times a day for 5 to 10 days were observed to have significantly greater weight gain (31% to 47%) compared to a control group receiving standard medical care. Explanations for this positive reaction include
- decreased levels of cortisol resulting in increased levels of oxytocin
- stimulation of the vagus nerve which extends from the cranium to the abdomen where it promotes the innervation of the viscera, enhances gastric motility, and increases release of hormones such as insulin which in turn increase nutrient absorption.

122. Web links:
a)*http://www.researchgate.net/researcher/9825743_Sari_Goldstein_Ferber*
b) *http://www.slideshare.net/MKayKeller/critical-review-8489403*
Journal: *Early Human Development, 37, 37-45.*
Title: Massage therapy by mothers and trained professionals enhances weight gain in preterm infants.
Authors: Ferber, S.G. Kuint, J., Weller, A., Feldman, R., Dollberg, S., Arbel, E., & Kohelet D. (2002).
Conclusions: For ten days, healthy preterm infants were divided into three groups. One, the control, received no massage therapy. Another group was massaged by female massage professionals. The third was massaged by their mothers. Those infants receiving massage from both professionals and mothers gained significantly more weight than those in the control group.

123. Web links:
 a) *http://www.researchgate.net/journal/0887-9311_Holistic_nursing_practice*
b) *http://journals.lww.com/hnpjournal/Abstract/2002/10000/Infant_Massage_as_a_Component_of_Developmental.4.aspx*
Journal: *Holistic Nursing Practice, 16, 1-7.*
Title: Infant massage as a component of developmental care: past, present, and future.
Authors: Mainous, R.O. (2002).

Conclusions: This study provides an overview of the use of infant massage. It has been used for centuries in parts of Africa, the Far East, and South America, but its use as a modality in North America is relatively new. Many studies have documented its efficacy with newborns in decreasing their stress levels, promoting weight gain, and improving motor function. Recent research has been conducted on the benefits of infant massage for those children with HIV, exposure to cocaine, and other illnesses.

124. Web link:
http://www.ncbi.nlm.nih.gov/pubmed/11677298
Journal: *Indian Pediatrics, 2001 Oct; 38(10):1091-8*
Title: Effects of tactile-kinesthetic stimulation on preterms: A controlled trial.
Authors: Mathai, S., Fernandez, A., Mondkar, J., & Kanbur, W. (2002).
Conclusions: 48 healthy preterm infants who weighed between 1000 and 2000 grams were assigned randomly to control and massage therapy groups. Those being massaged received infant massage and guided kinetic exercises from the third day of life to their term corrected age. In the hospital, their following vital parameters were observed:
- Oxygen saturation
- Temperature
- Heart rate
- Respiration

When they got home, they continued to receive the massage/kinetic therapy.
Compared to the control group, the massaged infants exhibited improved scores on the Brazelton scale on
- Autonomic stability
- Orientation
- Range of state
- Regulation of state

They also showed increased weight gain of 4.24 more grams per day than the controls and an increase in heart rate, within normal range.

125. Web link:
http://jpepsy.oxfordjournals.org/content/28/6/403.abstract
Journal: *Journal of Pediatric Psychology, 28, 403-411.*
Title: Stable preterm infants gain more weight and sleep less after five days of massage therapy.
Authors: Dieter, J., Field, T., Hernandez-Reif, M., Emory, E.K., & Redzepi, M. (2003).
Conclusions: Preterm babies who received five days of massage therapy gained 47% more weight than preterms who did not.

126. Web link:
<ins>http://www.articledashboard.com/Article/Massage-Therapy-and-Exercise-May-Improve-Bone-Mineralization-in-Premature-Infants-in-Marlboro-NJ/1184182</ins>

Journal: *Journal of Perinatology, 24, 305-309.*

Title: Physical activity combined with massage improves bone mineralization in the premature infants: A randomized trial.

Authors: Aly, H., Moustafa, M.F., Hassanein, S.M., Massaro, A.N., Amer, H.A., & Patel, K. (2004).

Conclusions: Premature infants suffer increased risk of mortality in part because of osteopenia, inability to form bones, and resorption of bones. In this study, thirty preterm neonates were divided into two groups, one a control and one which received massage and kinetic activity. The control group experienced decreased bone formation and increased bone resorption. The massage group experienced increased bone formation yet continued to have bone resorption as evidenced by Serum type I collagen C-terminal propeptide (PICP) and urinary pyridinoline crosslinks of collagen (Pyd) as indices.

Pulmonary Disease

127. Web link:
http://www.mendeley.com/research/effectiveness-acupressure-improving-dyspnoea-chronic-obstructive-pulmonary-disease-1/
Journal: *Journal of Advanced Nursing, 45, 252-259.*
Title: Effectiveness of acupressure in improving dyspnoea in chronic obstructive pulmonary disease [COPD].
Authors: Wu, H.S., Wu, S.C., Lin, J.G., & Lin, L.C. (2004).
Conclusions: 44 patients with COPD were divided into two groups. One was given acupressure at a true acupoint, the other to a sham acupoint. Both programs were five sessions a week for 4 weeks for a total of 20 treatments. Each session lasted 16 minutes. Before and after the program, both groups were measured on the Pulmonary Functional Status and Dyspnea Questionnaire-modified scale and the Spielberger State Anxiety scale and given a six minute walking test. Those in the true acupoint group showed significant improvement compared to those in the sham acupoint group.

Renal Disease

128. Web link:
http://www.mendeley.com/research/depression-symptoms-and-the-quality-of-life-in-patients-on-hemodialysis-for-endstage-renal-disease/
Journal: *Journal of Advanced Nursing (2003) Volume: 42, Issue: 2, Pp: 134-142*
Title: Acupoints massage in improving the quality of sleep and quality of life in patients with end-stage renal disease.
Authors: Tsay, S.L., Rong, J.R., & Lin, P.F. (2003)
Conclusions: Patients with end stage kidney disease have trouble sleeping and have a diminished quality of life. In this study, 98 patients were randomly assigned to one of three groups:
1. an acupressure group
2. a sham acupressure group
3. a control group

Compared to the control group, those in the acupuncture group slept better, longer, and with significantly decreased time waking as measured by the Pittsburgh Sleep Quality Index, Sleep Log, and the Medical Outcome Study – Short Form 36. These indices also documented that patients in the acupressure group had improved quality of life.

Respiratory Infections

129. Web link:
http://www.ncbi.nlm.nih.gov/pubmed/10453599
Journal: *J Tradit Chin Med. 1998 Dec;18(4):285-91.*
Title: A clinical investigation on massage for prevention and treatment of recurrent respiratory tract infection in children.
Authors: Zhu S, Wang N, Wang D, Wang M, Tong K, Xu H, Wang J, Li Q, Peng J, Wang J.
Conclusions: After three to six months of massage therapy on a group of healthy children and children susceptible to respiratory infection, it was found that massage produced a statistically significant benefit to those children massaged. All of their immunological indexes were about normal, their general constitution improved as did their immune functions. Massage was found to prevent and treat respiratory conditions.

Restless Leg Syndrome

130. Web link:
http://www.sciencedirect.com/science/article/pii/S1360859206001483
Journal: *Journal of Bodywork and Movement Therapies Volume 11, Issue 2, April 2007, Pages 146-150*
Title: Massage therapy and restless legs syndrome
Author: Meg Russell LMBT[1]

Conclusions: This paper is a case study on the effects of massage therapy done on a 35 year old woman suffering from Restless Leg Syndrome (RLS). The following modalities were used twice weekly for three weeks in a 45 minute massage to the leg, focusing on the hamstring and piriformis muscles:
- myofascial release
- trigger point therapy
- deep tissue
- sports massage techniques

Before, during, and after the study, the patient completed a Functional Rating index assessing her intensity level, frequency, and duration of RLS symptoms, and she also kept a log of hours slept, nocturnal waking, intensity and manner of RLS symptoms, intake of stimulants and medications, and level of stress. The patient's symptoms of sleeplessness, urge to move legs, and tingling sensations all decreased after just the first two treatments and continued to improve for the rest of the three week study.

Rheumatoid Arthritis

131. Web link:
http://jpepsy.oxfordjournals.org/content/22/5/607.full.pdf
Journal: *Journal of Pediatric Psychology, Vol. 22, No. 5, 1997, pp. 607-617*
Title: Juvenile Rheumatoid Arthritis: Benefits from Massage Therapy
Authors: Tiffany Field, Maria Hernandez-Reif, Susan Seligman,
Josh Krasnegor, and William Sunshine
Conclusions: 20 children with JRA were divided into two groups. One received 15 minutes of massage per day from their parents for 30 days, first in the supine position, then in the prone position. The other group was engaged in relaxation therapy. A pediatric rheumatologist assessed the children before and after the sessions on the first and last days of the 30-day study using the following:
- The State Anxiety Inventory (STAI; Spielberger, Gorsuch, & Lushene,1970)
- Behavior Observation of the Child's Anxiety Level to assess behavior following relaxation therapy classes
- Cortisol Samples.

The neurologist determined that those children in the massage group had significantly lower levels of stress, anxiety, cortisol, and pain compared to the relaxation group.

132. Web link: *http://itandb.com/pdf/arthritis-massage.pdf*
Journal: *Journal of Bodywork and Movement Therapies (2007) 11, 21–24*
Title: Hand arthritis pain is reduced by massage therapy
Authors: Tiffany Field, Miguel Diego, Maria Hernandez-Reif, Jean Shea
Conclusions: Researchers from the University of Miami School of Medicine randomly assigned twenty adult patients with rheumatoid arthritis of the wrist and hand either for massage therapy or to a control group. Those in the massage group received therapy once a week for four weeks and were taught to massage the afflicted hand/wrist daily at home. Compared to the control group those patients doing massage showed lower levels of anxiety and depression, less pain, and greater grip strength.

Rotator Cuff Injuries

133. Web link:
http://www.pcc.edu/library/news/prize/conservative_treatment.pdf
Journal: *unpublished research paper presented to Dr. Consuelo Romanski, Ph.D.*
Title: Conservative Treatment of Rotator Cuff Injuries to Avoid Surgical Repair
Authors: Jill Schuldt, LMT

Conclusions: The author reviews research studies, clinical findings, and experimental data to conclude that for those with rotator cuff injuries without tears, conservative treatment with massage therapy results in
- Pain reduction
- Increased flexibility
- But no increase in strength

For those with tears, although the tears may not heal, they often become symptom free with massage and without the need for surgery. If after six months of conservative treatment with massage there is insufficient improvement, then surgery is indicated.

Sexual Abuse

134. Web link: *http://www6.miami.edu/touch-research/AdultMassage.html*
Journal: *Journal of Bodywork and Movement Therapies, 1, 65-69.*
Title: Sexual abuse effects are lessened by massage therapy.
Authors: Field, T., Hernandez-Reif, M., Hart, S., Quintino, O., Drose, L., Field, T., Kuhn, C., & Schanberg, S. (1997).
Conclusions: This study evaluated whether women who had been sexually abused (mean age 35) would benefit from massage therapy compared to a control group which underwent relaxation techniques. They were given massage twice a week for one month. Following each of

their sessions they reported less anxiety and depression, and their salivary cortisol levels dropped. After one month, both groups reported decreases in depression and anxiety, but the massage group showed decreases in stress hormone levels and in life event stress, whereas the relaxation group had increasingly negative feelings about being touched.

Sleep

135. Web link:
http://www.ncbi.nlm.nih.gov/pubmed/20056221
Journal: Int J Nurs Stud. 2010 Jul;47(7):798-805. Epub 2010 Jan 6.
Title: "Effectiveness of acupressure for residents of long-term care facilities with insomnia: A randomized controlled trial,"
Authors: Sun JL, Sung MS, Huang MY, Cheng GC, Lin CC.

Conclusions: Fifty residents of two long term health care facilities in Taiwan were divided into a control group or were treated with acupressure at point Heart 7 for insomnia over a six week period. From weeks three to six, none of the patients in the acupressure group reported any insomnia! The study concluded that "Acupressure on the HT7 point may improve insomnia for up to 2 weeks after the intervention."

136. Web link:

http://ajcc.aacnjournals.org/content/7/4/288.abstract

Journal: *American Journal of Critical Care, 7,* 288-299.

critically ill patients.

Authors: Richards, K.C. (1998).

Conclusions: Critically ill patients often have difficulty sleeping which impairs their recuperation [anabolism occurs during periods of sleep]. Nonpharmacological techniques to assist sleep had never been evaluated before this study which assessed the efficacy of the following methods on a random assortment of 69 critically ill men:

1. back massage
2. a combination of muscle relaxation, mental imagery, and a music audiotape
3. normal nursing care

Only those in the back massage group showed statistically significant evidence of improvement of quality of sleep.

Smoking

137. Web link:

http://www.massagetherapycanada.com/content/view/1371/38/

Journal: *Preventive Medicine, 28,* 28-32.

Title: Smoking cravings are reduced by self-massage.

Authors: Hernandez-Reif, M., Field, T., & Hart, S. (1999).

Conclusions: In a study of twenty smokers assigned to either a massage therapy group or a control group, those receiving massages were taught to do self massage to their hands or ears three times a day for a month. By the last week of the study, those in the massage group were smoking fewer cigarettes per day than those in the control group. They also reported less withdrawal symptoms, less anxiety, and improved mood.

Spinal Cord Injuries

138. Web link:
http://www.ncbi.nlm.nih.gov/pubmed/12325402
Journal: *International Journal of Neuroscience, 112*, 133-142.
Title: Spinal cord patients benefit from massage therapy.
Authors: Diego, M.A., Field, T., Hernandez-Reif, M., Hart, S., Brucker, B., Field, Tory, Burman, I. (2002).
Conclusions: Twenty patients who had received spinal cord injuries to vertebrae C5 through C7 were randomly assigned either to an exercise group or to a massage therapy group. For five weeks, those in the massage group received a 40 minute massage twice a week. Patients in the exercise group targeted their arms, back, neck, and shoulders with range of motion exercises twice weekly for five weeks. Both groups benefited, but only the massage group demonstrated:
- lower levels of anxiety
- lower levels of depression
- significantly greater range of motion in the wrist

- significantly greater muscle strength

Stress

139. Web link:
http://www.mendeley.com/research/endocrinological-evaluations-of-brief-hand-massages-in-palliative-care/
Journal: *Journal of Alternative and Complementary Medicine, 15,* 981-985.
Title: Endocrinological evaluations of brief hand massages in palliative care.
Authors: Osaka, I., Kurihara, Y., Tanaka, K., Nishizaki, H., Aoki, S., Adachi, I. (2009).
Conclusions: In this study, 34 terminally ill cancer patients were treated with a 5 minute massage to the hands. Saliva was collected from each patient before and after the massage to assess levels of chromogranin A (CgA), a biomarker for levels of stress. The brief massage did result in reduced levels of chromogranin A (CgA), indicating reduced levels of stress, and a statistically significant number of patients reported satisfaction with the experience.

Stroke

140. Web link:
http://www.sciencedirect.com/science/article/pii/S1353611704000423
Journal: *Complementary Therapies of Nursing Midwifery, 10, 209-216.*
Title: The effects of slow-stroke back massage on anxiety and shoulder pain in elderly stroke patients.
Authors: Mok, E., & Woo, C.P. (2004).
Conclusions: Slow stroke back massage (SSBM) was performed for 10 minutes seven evenings in a row on 102 elderly patients who had suffered a stroke and been hospitalized. The group consisted of 102 patients who were split into two groups, one being massaged and the other a control. The two groups were evaluated for heart rate, blood pressure, and self-reported levels of anxiety and pain. Findings were that in the SSBM group there were significantly lower levels of pain and anxiety. Also, patients in the SSBM group relaxed as evidenced objectively by lower levels of systolic and diastolic blood pressure and heart rate. These benefits persisted for three days after the massages, and the patients felt positively about SSBM.

Surgery

141. Web link:
http://www.sciencedirect.com/science/article/pii/S0886335000007306
Journal: *Journal of Cataract & Refractive Surgery, 27, 884-890.*
Title: Effects of hand massage on anxiety in cataract surgery using local anesthesia.
Authors: Kim, M.S., Cho, K.S., Woo, H., & Kim, J.H. (2001).
Conclusions: Patients undergoing surgery experience anxiety, and this can be quantified by measuring blood pressure; heart rate; levels of epinephrine, norepinephrine, blood sugar, cortisol, lymphocytes, and neutrophils; and using the Visual Analog Scale. This study employed those measurements on 59 patients before and after having cataract surgery. They were divided into two groups – a control and those having 5 minutes of hand massage before surgery. Five minutes after surgery, those in the control group had elevated levels of epinephrine, norepinephrine, and cortisol – all signs of increased anxiety. However, those levels did not increase for patients in the massage group, and all other indices of anxiety decreased in the massage group.

142. Web link:
http://www.ahhthatsthespotmassage.com/medicalmassageinfo.asp
Journal: *Likarska Sprava, 93-96.*
Title: Effect of neck massage therapy on the soft tissues after thyroid surgery.
Authors: Antoniv, V.R. (2002)
Conclusions: After thyroid surgery, patients were given neck massage to improve skin and muscle tone of the neck. In 85% of cases there was improvement. Also, 48% of patients reported reduced swelling and edema.

Tennis Elbow

143. Web link: *http://ptjournal.apta.org/content/83/7/608*
Journal: *Physical Therapy, October 2011, Volume 91, Issue 10*
Title: Manipulation of the Wrist for Management of Lateral Epicondylitis: A Randomized Pilot Study
Authors: Twenty-eight patients with lateral epicondylitis were assigned to one of two groups:
1. This group received manipulation of the wrist.
2. This group received friction massage, muscle stretching, and ultrasound.

After three weeks patients in Group 1 had a 62% success rate compared to 20% for those in Group 2. After six weeks, on a pain scale of 1 to 11 patients in Group 1 reported an improvement in pain of 5.2 versus 3.2 in Group 2.

Manipulation of the wrist appeared to be the more effective therapy.

Thumb and Trigger Finger Pain

144. Web link:
http://www.ncbi.nlm.nih.gov/pmc/articles/PMC1864591/
Journal: *J Can Chiropr Assoc. 2006 December; 50(4): 249–254.*
Title: The conservative treatment of Trigger Thumb using Graston Techniques and Active Release Techniques®
Authors: Scott Howitt, DC, FCCSS(C), FCCRS(C),[*] Jerome Wong, DC, and Sonja Zabukovec, DC
Conclusions: This is a case study of the treatment of one patient with trigger thumb ("fibrocartilagenous metaplasia and hypertrophy of the surrounding structures of the flexor tendon resulting in a painful and debilitating restriction of motion") using the Graston Technique®, which involves augmenting soft tissue mobilization with stainless steel instruments used in a stroking motion applied to the skin at a 30-60 degree angle. This enables the clinician to detect abnormalities in the underlying soft tissue, remove scar tissue adhesions, and enhance the proliferation of fibroblasts. Active Release Techniques (ART) were also used to remove adhesions and promote normal soft tissue growth. This patient was relieved of his pain and had increased range of motion after having eight treatments of Active Release Techniques® and Graston technique.

TMJ

145. Web link:
http://www.ncbi.nlm.nih.gov/pubmed/14520768
Journal: *J Orofac Pain. 2003 Summer;17(3):224-36.*
Title: Use of complementary and alternative medicine for temporomandibular disorders.
Authors: DeBar LL, Vuckovic N, Schneider J, Ritenbaugh C.
Conclusions: 192 patients with TMJ were surveyed to see if they used complementary and alternative methods to treat the disorder. 120 reported yes, and of that number, massage therapy was the most commonly used and reported to be the most effective.

Torticollis

146. Web link: *http://eng.hi138.com/?i149689*
Journal: *Free Papers Download Center*
Title: Massage treatment of children with muscular torticollis in 32 cases of clinical experience
Authors: unknown
Conclusions: A group of 32 infants ranging in ages from 20 days to 18 months with muscular torticollis were treated with massage to relieve the condition. There were 18 males and 14 females. The children were treated in a sitting or lying position, and to prevent skin damage, talc was used as a lubricant. The following massage techniques were employed:

- (1) Anrou law: the doctor rubbed the affected side with the thumb pulp at the Feng-chi point (Gall Bladder 20), and then from the top down along the sternocleidomastoid muscle. This was repeated several times, focusing on the local mass.
- (2) The doctor placed his/her thumb on the tumor (muscle mass) and repeatedly plucked the surrounding tissue. This was repeated 3 to 5 times.
- (3) Traction rotation law: the doctor put one hand on the ipsilateral or affected side shoulder and one hand on the ispilateral head and gradually stretched the contralateral head and shoulder. Then the doctor gradually lengthened the mastoid ipsilateral sternoclavicular muscle, ranging from small mounting. Then the doctor rotated the head to the ipsilateral side 5 to 10 times.
- (4) The doctor used the thumb to press on the ipsilateral shoulder a few times, and then used the hypothenar eminence of the thumb to press the shoulder and neck and finally pushed at acupressure points Stomach 12 and Gall Bladder 21.

Transplants

147. Web link:
http://www.intelihealth.com/IH/ihtIH/WSIHW000/8513/34968/358873.html?d=dmtContent
Journal: Alternative Therapies, 9, 40-49.
Title: Outcomes of touch therapies during bone marrow transplant.
Authors: Smith, M.C., Reeder, F., Daniel, L., Baramee, J., & Hagman, J. (2003).
Conclusions: Compared to a control group, 58 patients receiving bone marrow transplants who received massage therapy or therapeutic touch every third day starting with the commencement of chemotherapy until discharge from the program showed significantly lower amounts of central nervous system or neurological complications. However no benefit was noted from among ten other categories of possible complications.

Vagal Activity

148. Web link:
http://www.jstage.jst.go.jp/article/biomedres/29/6/29_317/_article
Journal: Biomedical Research, 29, 317-320.
Title: Facial massage reduced anxiety and negative mood status, and increased sympathetic nervous activity.
Authors: Hatayama, T., Kitamura, S., Tamura, C., Nagano, M., & Ohnuki, K. (2008).

Conclusions: Thirty-two healthy women were treated with a 45 minute facial massage to evaluate the effects on their autonomic nervous systems, mood, and level of anxiety via an assessment of heart rate variability (HRV) with spectral analysis. The State Trait Anxiety Inventory (STAI) and the Profile of Mood Status (POMS) were also given to determine psychological status, and both were significantly reduced after the massage. The low to high frequency ratio (LF/HF ratio) of heart rate variability was also lowered. Researchers concluded that facial massage reduced psychological distress and activated the sympathetic nervous system and might thereby refresh the patients.

Voice Disorders

149. Web link:
http://www.ingentaconnect.com/content/apl/slog/2000/00 000025/00000004/art00002
Journal: *Logopedics, Phoniatrics, Vocology, 25, 146-150.*
Title: An effect of body massage on voice loudness and phonation frequency in reading.
Authors: Ternstrom, S., Andersson, M., & Bergman, U. (2000).
Conclusions: Researchers investigated the effect of massage on the fundamental frequency of the voice and sound pressure level. Thirty-one patients were recorded reading a 3 minute passage of prose from a book. Sixteen patients were then massaged for 30 minutes

while 15 control subjects rested. Thereafter both groups were asked to read the same 3 minute passage from a book. Those in the massage group evidenced lower fundamental frequency and sound pressure level.

Whiplash – Mechanical Neck Disorders

150. Web link:
http://journals.lww.com/spinejournal/Abstract/2007/02010/Massage_for_Mechanical_Neck_Disorders__A.12.aspx
Journal: *Spine: 1 February 2007 - Volume 32 - Issue 3 - pp 353-362*
Title: Massage for Mechanical Neck Disorders: A Systematic Review
Authors: Ezzo, Jeanette PhD, CMT; Haraldsson, Bodhi G. RMT; Gross, Anita R. MSc; Myers, Cynthia D. PhD, LMT; Morien, Annie PhD, PA-C, LMT; Goldsmith, Charlie H. PhD; Bronfort, Gert PhD, DC; Peloso, Paul M. MD, MSc
Conclusions: This study provides an overview of the results of 19 studies on the use of massage for whiplash and mechanical disorders of the neck. The researchers noted that massage is often used for the treatment of neck pain, but 12 of the 19 studies were poorly designed and not useful for determining the efficacy of massage. Six studies examined massage as a treatment by itself, not used in conjunction with other therapies, but the results were inconclusive. In 14 studies in which massage was used along with other therapies, the study

designs were flawed in that one could not assess how much massage contributed to the patient's recovery as apart from the other therapies. Thus no recommendations could be made, except that further studies are needed which specify the frequency of massage treatments, their duration, number of sessions, and specific technique employed.

Afterword

You know medical paradigms are changing when the conservative **Wall Street Journal** writes that massage "has a wide variety of tangible health benefits" as it did March 13, 2012 in a feature article entitled "Don't Call It Pampering: Massage Wants to Be Medicine."

The article refers to many of the studies cited in this book and notes that "The American College of Physicians and the American Pain Society now include massage as one of their recommendations for treating low back pain." It's about time.

Massage research at the National Center for Complementary and Alternative Medicine (NCCAM) is now up to $2.7 million. By comparison NCCAM's parent organization, the National Institutes of Health, spent $32.1 billion – yes, billion – on medical research in 2011. When one considers that 8.3% of the American population spent $11 billion for massage therapy in 2007, it is apparent that massage is getting short-changed both in terms of research funding and respect by the medical establishment.

In 2010 Americans spent $2.6 trillion on health care, and David Walker, formerly Comptroller General of the U.S. observed that future unfunded government liabilities for Medicare amount to $36.3 Trillion. Yes - $36.3 Trillion, with a "T." It'll take a major miracle to resolve that financial crisis.

The purpose of massage therapy is to empower the body to get well on its own, not to foster a lifelong dependency on drugs or surgical procedures. Massage is enjoyable, effective without side effects, and inexpensive – often much less expensive the Medicare approved medical procedures. Ironically, many of Jesus' healing miracles from 2,000 years ago involved His use of touch. Is there anything to be learned from that example?

About the Authors

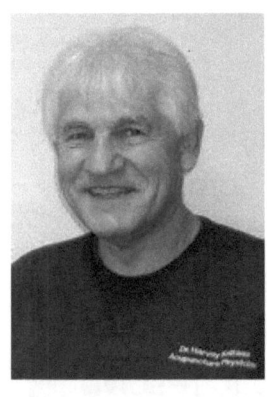 Dr. Harvey Kaltsas, Acupuncture Physician, is a graduate of Williston Academy ('65) and Amherst College ('69), an alumnus of Boston University School of Law ('72) and the North American College of Acupuncture ('75), and a graduate of the New England School of Acupuncture ('77). Since apprenticing with Drs. John Ho Fen Shen and James Tin Yau So, he has been practicing acupuncture and Oriental medicine for 36 years.

Dr. Kaltsas has been President of the Florida State Acupuncture Association and the American Association of Acupuncture and

Oriental Medicine (AAAOM); and as Chair of the Florida Board of Acupuncture he co-wrote most of the regulations governing the practice of acupuncture in Florida. In 1993 he was commended by the People's Republic of China for his contributions to the field of acupuncture, and in 1996 he was named Acupuncturist of the year by AAAOM. He is the only acupuncturist ever to deliver testimony regarding acupuncture to the US Senate (June, 1993), and in 2008-9 he served as Legislative Chair for AAAOM and as official liaison to AAAOM's lobbyist in Washington, D.C.

For the past four years Dr. Kaltsas has served as visiting acupuncturist at the annual conferences of the National Foundation for Women Legislators. He is in private practice in Sarasota, Florida and has recently authored Acupuncture Works – the Proof, a compendium of 157 peer-reviewed studies documenting the cost-effectiveness of acupuncture. He was co-founder of Sarasota's Academy of Chinese Healing Arts (since renamed East West College) and now teaches 15 nationally approved Continuing Education courses online at www.hkacup.com .

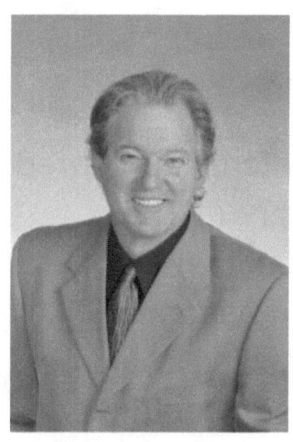

Butch Phelps is a Florida Licensed Massage Therapist, is a graduate of The Florida College of Natural Health(2005), Personal Trainer since 1996, certified in Active Isolated Stretching(2006) and awarded Distinguished Toastmasters award(2011), the highest honor given to a Toastmasters. Butch studied with Aaron Mattes, founder of Active Isolated Stretching(2006).

Butch Phelps was awarded the Golden Hands Award from The Florida College of Natural Health. This award is given by the teachers of that school. Butch owns The Muscle Repair

Shop, 2009 Greater Sarasota Chamber of Commerce "Young Business of the Year."

Since graduation from school, Butch volunteered one afternoon a week for five years at The Senior Friendship Center in Sarasota, Florida, to better understand how effective massage therapy and Active Isolated Stretching could be for seniors. Upon leaving the senior center, Butch had a waiting lists for more than 60 days in advance.

Butch has worked with athletes of all levels, children, and patients with major disabilities.

Since 2008, Butch has been a District leader in Toastmasters International, earned his Distinguished Toastmasters Designation, and competed in several speaking contests. Butch has given many speeches to universities, organizations, and businesses. Butch is available for speaking engagements. To contact Butch you can call 941-922-2929 or email him at butch@musclerepairshop.com.

To learn more please go to
www.musclerepairshop.com.

www.ingramcontent.com/pod-product-compliance
Lightning Source LLC
Chambersburg PA
CBHW030814180526
45163CB00003B/1276